Who looks outside, dreams; who looks inside awakens.

carl jung

Contents
Issue 09

Publishers
Justin Faerman
Meghan McDonald

Editors
Justin Faerman
Meghan McDonald

Copy Editors
Meghan McDonald
Shari Hollander

Art Director
Justin Faerman

Designer
Justin Faerman

Visit Us On The Web
consciouslifestylemag.com

Conscious Lifestyle Magazine
is published four times yearly. Subscriptions can be purchased through our website listed below or through Apple Newsstand via the iTunes Store. All rights reserved. No part of this publication may be used without written permission from the publishers. The publishers expressly disclaim all liability for any occurrence that may arise as a consequence of the use of the information presented in this magazine.

© 2015
Conscious Lifestyle Magazine

Cover Photo
Adam Kay

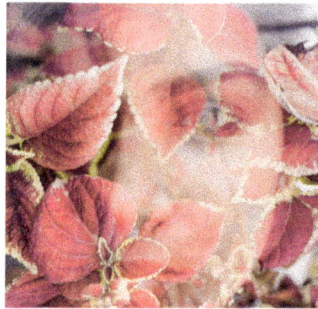
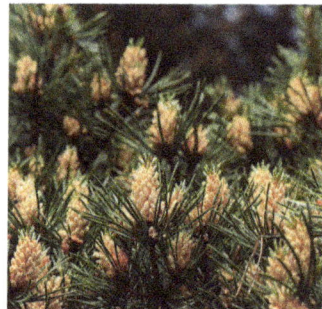
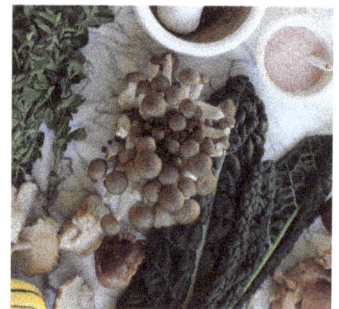
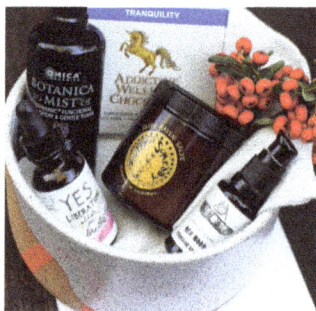
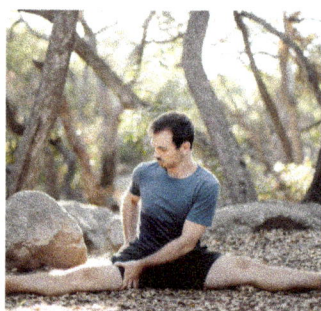
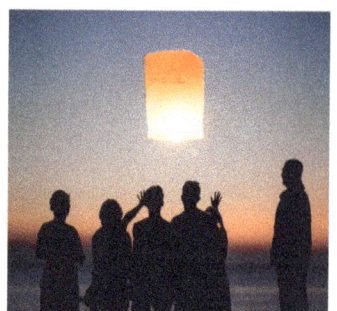

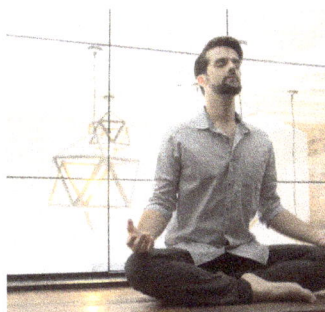

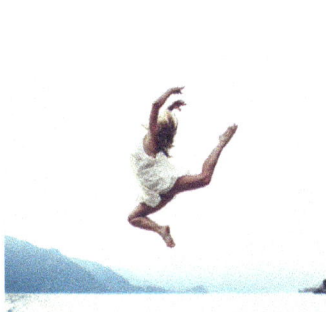

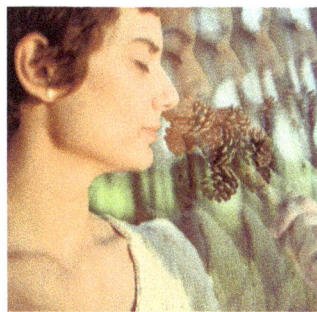

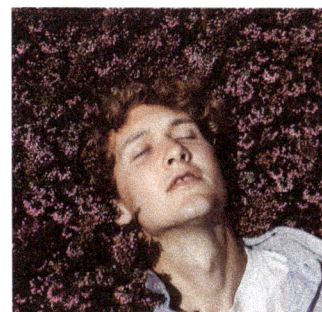

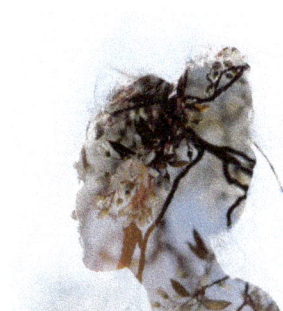

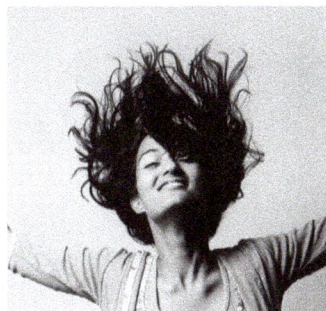

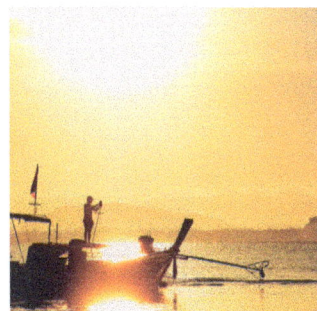

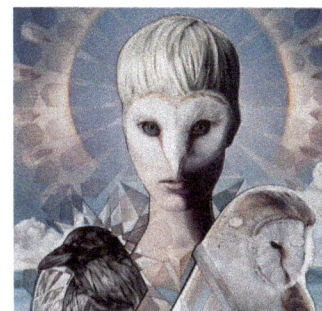

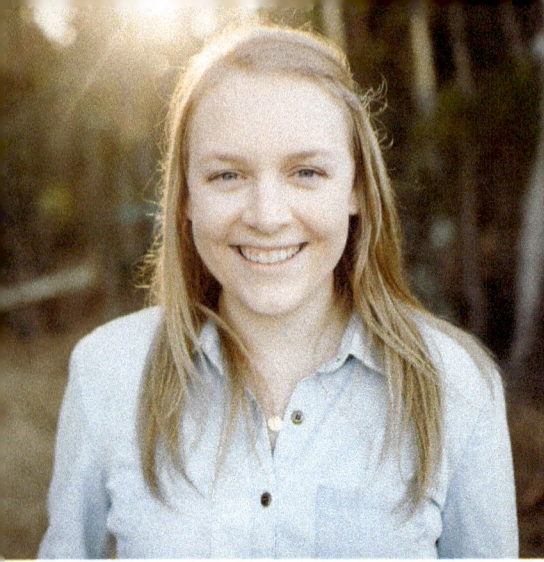

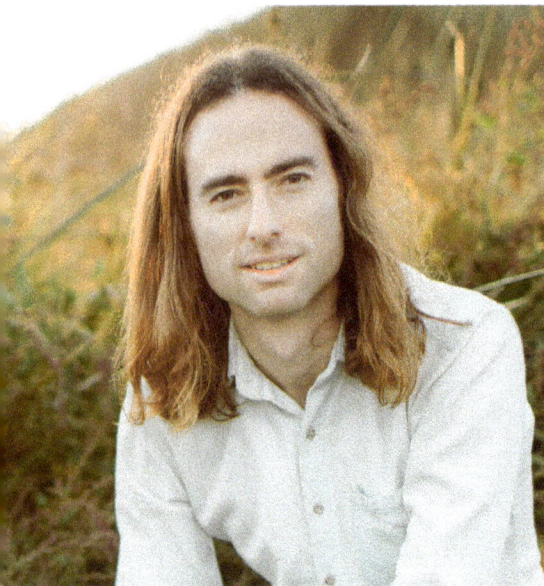

LETTER FROM THE EDITORS

Over the last few months it is as if the cosmos are quietly whispering to us: "Let go of the way you think things should be and trust the infinitely wise unfolding that is occurring in every moment."

As Eckhart Tolle is so fond of saying "Life will give you whatever experience is most helpful for the evolution of your consciousness. How do you know this is the experience you need? Because this is the experience you are having at the moment."

And they are both right—he and the cosmos, that is. Although we humans like to think otherwise, everything is unfolding with a perfectness and precision that is so intricate and immense that we perceive it as chaos. Let that sink in for a moment, because the implications are vast. We live in a universe of perfect balance and synchrony, although this truth is often lost within the distorted perceptions of the human mind—one that is serving up in real time an infinite number of simultaneous realities and experiences uniquely tailored to each splinter of consciousness, from the tiniest cells to the towering elephants and every single thing in between, in a never ending dance of growth, expansion, and evolution.

The good, the bad, the ugly... all of it with a purpose to ultimately enlighten, to help consciousness know itself, to have the experience of separation so that we may know oneness. To have the experience of transgression so we may know forgiveness. And with the understanding of this truth we are free to let go and trust the wisdom of life, a theme we will explore throughout this issue in the hopes that it may bring you more freedom, joy and peace.

justin faerman + meghan mcdonald
Co-founders, Conscious Lifestyle Magazine

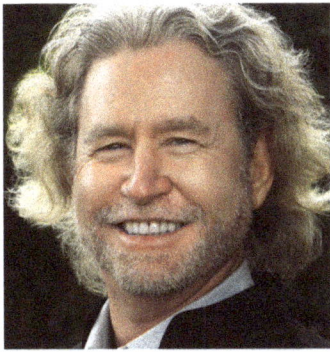

Ronald Alexander Ph.D.

is a mind-body psychotherapist, international leadership consultant, and the Executive Director of the OpenMind Training Institute in Santa Monica, a leading-edge organization that offers personal and professional training programs in mind-body therapies, transformational leadership, and mindfulness. He is the author of the widely acclaimed book *Wise Mind, Open Mind* that provides practical and innovative applications to help us through challenging times. Visit his website: *ronaldalexander.com*

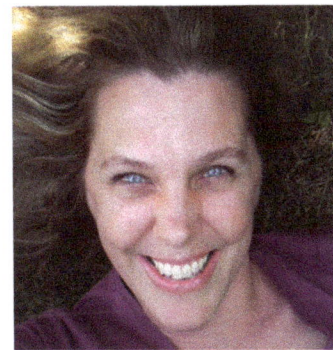

Cynthia Sue Larson

is a best-selling author and life coach who helps talented people struggling with unsatisfying lives find love, meaning, and prosperity. Cynthia has a degree in physics from UC Berkeley, and practices and teaches meditation and mar-

tial arts. She has been featured on numerous shows including the History Channel, Coast to Coast AM, and the BBC. Endorsed by Dr. Larry Dossey, Fred Alan Wolf, and Stanley Krippner, her newest book, *Quantum Jumps*, describes the science of instantaneous transformation emerging from the convergence of recent research findings in physics, biology, and psychology. Vist her website: *realityshifters.com*

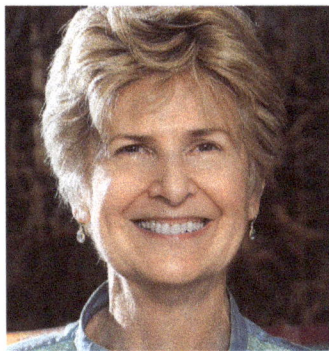

Katie Hendricks Ph.D.

is passionate about the power of embodied integrity and emergence and continuously promotes creative expression in service of a direct experience of life, wholeness and evolutionary collaboration. She has been a pioneer in the field of body-mind integration for over 40 years. Katie has an international reputation as a seminar leader, training professionals from many fields in the core skills of conscious living through the lens of body intelligence. Katie earned a Ph.D. in transpersonal psychology and has been a Board Certified-Dance/Movement Therapist since 1975. Visit her website: *hendricks.com*

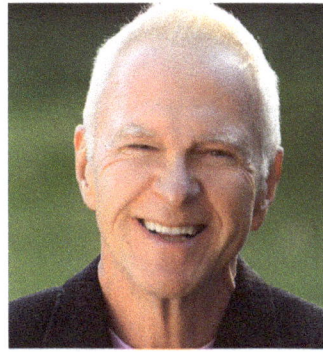

Gay Hendricks Ph.D.

has been a leader in the fields of relationship transformation and body-mind therapies for over 45 years. After earning his Ph.D. in counseling psychology from Stanford, Gay served as professor of counseling psychology at the University of Colorado for 21 years. He has written and co-authored (with Katie) 35 books, including the bestseller *Conscious Loving*. Gay has offered seminars worldwide and appeared on more than 500 radio and television shows, including *Oprah, CNN, CNBC, 48 Hours* and others. Visit his website: *hendricks.com*

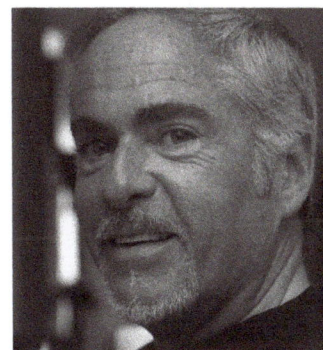

Mark Mincolla Ph.D.

is a legendary natural health care practitioner who has transformed the lives of many thousands of people over the past 30 years. He

dream as if you'll live forever. live as if you'll die tomorrow.

unknown

has ingeniously integrated ancient Chinese energy techniques with cutting-edge nutritional science in his innovative Electromagnetic Muscle Testing (EMT) system. Mark brings his 30 years of experience as a natural health expert to millions of television viewers and talk radio listeners throughout New England and the nation each week, sharing cutting edge nutrition and natural health information to help followers take control of their lives so that they might better preserve their precious health. He maintains a personal practice in Cohasset, Massachusetts, where he lives. Visit his website: *markmincolla.com*

most obstacles melt away when we make up our minds to walk boldly through them.

unknown

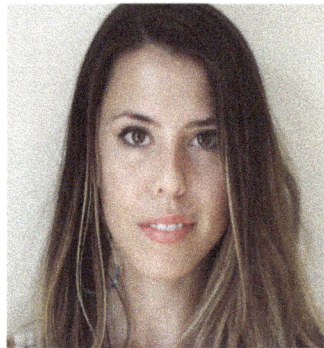

Claire Ragozzino

is a certified yoga instructor, plant-based chef, and holistic wellness educator. Blending Ayurvedic principles, plant-based nutrition, and yogic philosophy to cultivate deep inner wisdom for intuitive healing, Claire works with clients around the globe to inspire transformational changes in their health and wellbeing. She is a resource for women looking to reconnect with their roots and the ancient wisdom of self-healing through food, breath, and conscious movement. Visit her website: *vidyaliving.com*

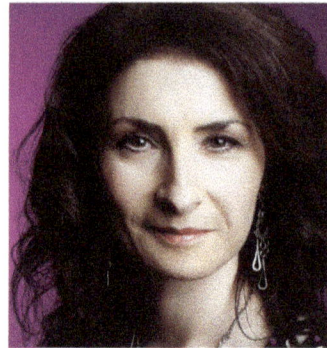

Julia McCutchen

is an intuitive mentor, the founder and creative director of the International Association of Conscious & Creative Writers (IACCW), and the author of *Conscious Writing: Discover Your True Voice Through Mindfulness and More*. A former publisher of spiritual and personal development books, a life-changing accident triggered a series of major quantum leaps in her spiritual awakening. Today, Julia's passion is to guide you to discover your true self and express your true voice on the page and in the world. Visit her websites: *JuliaMcCutchen.com* and *iaccw.com*

Donna Stoneham, Ph.D.

is an executive coach, transformational leadership consultant, and educator, helping

hundreds of Fortune 1000 and not-for-profit leaders, teams, and organizations "unleash their power to thrive™" through her company, Positive Impact, LLC. Dr. Stoneham has written for the *International Journal of Coaches in Organizations* and *Presence*, is a certified Integral Coach®, and is a popular speaker and media guest. When she's not coaching, she enjoys swimming, traveling, writing, and spending time at home with her spouse and rescue dogs. Visit her website: *donnastoneham.com*

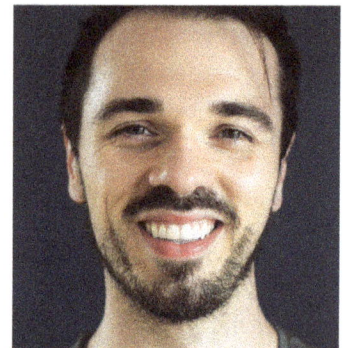

Matt Cooke

is a neuroscience-based yoga teacher (500 RYT), author, and High Performance Coach who uses movement to unleash high performance for burnt out tech entrepreneurs. Matt studied extensively with Noah Maze and Elena Brower and his work is infused with Kripalu, Iyengar, and several coaching methodologies. Having conducted workshops and seminars all over the world, Matt is impassioned to inspire action and embodiment off the yoga mat. To learn more about Matt or get in touch with him, visit his website: *mattcooke.yoga*

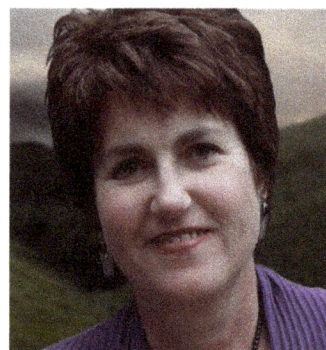

Alexa Gray

is a passionate health coach, wellness educator, and natural health writer committed to teaching practical tools for ultimate wellbeing. Through her colorful blog SuperFood SuperLife, she shares great products, restaurants, artisans and literature that are close to nature, made with compassion, and revitalize the spirit. A trained fine art photographer based in L.A., Alexa is also a certified holistic health practitioner and certified raw foods nutritionist. She is currently creating creative content for other companies and consulting brands as a freelance social media strategist. Visit her website: *superfoodsuperlife.com*

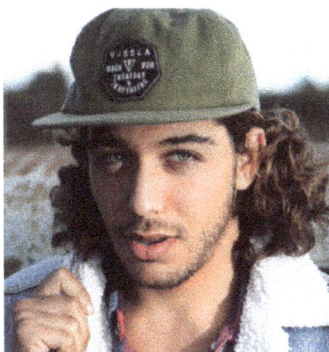

Collin Elder

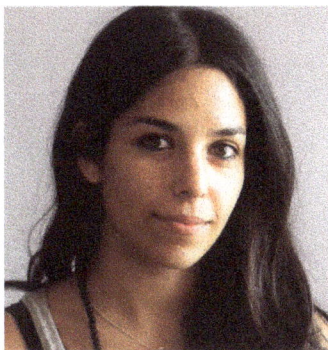

began painting after leaving the realm of ecological conservation, which, along with a degree in wildlife biology, has focused his artwork on our deep and often mysterious connections with the natural world. His paintings reflect a yearning to further pursue the depths of our links with the non-human, and hopefully connect the remembering of them with the health of our human community. Visit his website: *collinelder.com*

Ryan Mandell

is a writer, musician, surfer, yogi, and artist. He developed an early interest in spirituality as a child finding himself strongly drawn to the eastern religions of Buddhism and Hinduism. After spending many years practicing yoga and studying the sutras, he began to find a deeper sense of his place in the collective conscious. His writing and art focus on the beauty of humanity, but do not hesitate to acknowledge its shadows and the places that need healing. Listen to his music at *getatpookie.bandcamp.com*

the real meditation is how you live your life.

jon kabat-zinn

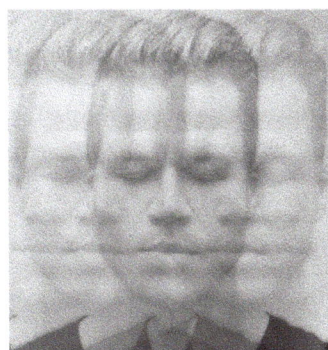

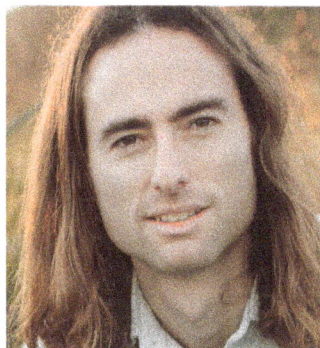

Justin Faerman

is a visionary change-agent, entrepreneur and healer dedicated to evolving global consciousness, bridging science and spirituality and spreading enlightened ideas on both an individual and societal level. He is the co-founder of Conscious Lifestyle Magazine and a sought after coach and teacher, known for his pioneering work in the area of flow. He is largely focused on applied spirituality, which is translating abstract spiritual concepts and ideas into practical, actionable techniques for creating a deeply fulfilling, prosperous life. Connect with him at *artofflowcoaching.com*

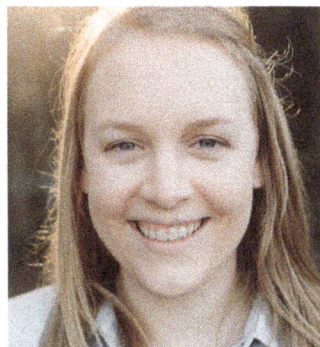

Meghan McDonald

is the co-founder and co-editor of Conscious Lifestyle Magazine. She holds a Masters degree in social psychology and has conducted award-winning research into the nature of human social behavoir.

the task ahead of you is never greater than the strength within you.

joseph campbell

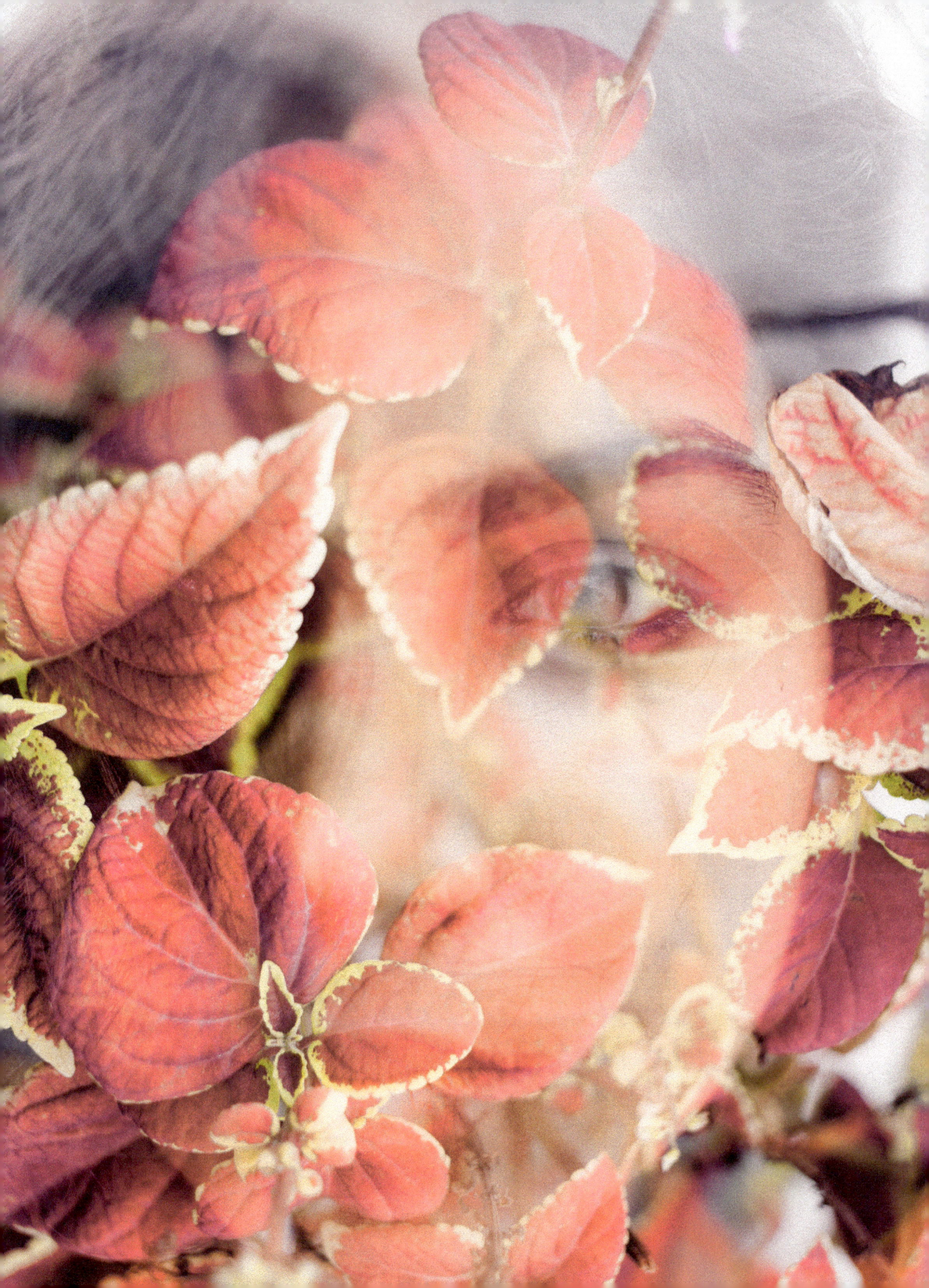

BIO-ENERGETICS

THE ART AND SCIENCE OF HARMONIZING YOUR MIND, BODY & SPIRIT

According to ancient Chinese medical wisdom, living in alignment with our unique energetic constitution is the key to radiant health

by mark mincolla, ph.d.

A code is a specialized language that trans-lates specific, unique information. One of the greatest examples of this is our genetic code, the language that defines and disseminates the unique information contained within our DNA. Similarly, Whole Health asserts that we each possess our own personal energy codes that can be broken down into a language, which represents all the unique information that makes us who and what we truly are. Whole Health refers to these exclusive energy codes as our constitution.

I recently enjoyed an interesting conversation with a pediatric nurse regarding human constitutions. We chatted for a few moments about my writing this piece. Our discussion immediately moved into the area of human variation. As we spoke, we drifted off a bit onto the topic of reincarnation. I questioned whether he believed in it and, if so, whether he felt it might play a role in the uniqueness of our constitutions. He said that

after more than a decade of attending to the birth of "preemies"—premature babies—he was inclined to believe that every single one had come into this world with a fully developed and unique inner core. He said that to his way of thinking, when it comes to the question of nature versus nurture, it was all about nature. He went on to further emphasize how, when you look into their eyes, each preemie reveals a separate, secret universe. As we parted, I reflected on the paradox of energy: how unique yet similar everything is.

I've often thought about the sense of oneness that orbiting astronauts must feel as they gaze down upon Mother Earth from miles up in space. From their lofty macrocosmic perspective, the galaxy appears as a holograph. Observing life at a quantum level, however, provides a glimpse of a world of tiny particles telling a completely different story about the profound uniqueness of all things that are as one. The way of energy is undivided yet *sui*

No one nutritional supplement, drug, or food can be good for everyone.

Science is beginning to find constitutionality showing up in the most unexpected places.

generis.

We are all as unique as the droplets that make up the same sea of energy. Separation is an illusion, yet the multiverse's varied manifestations remain but a reflection of its unanimity and flux. Even though we are constituents of the same sea, your energy is different from mine. Our energy is different today than it was yesterday, and it will continue to change throughout the course of any given moment, day, week, month, and year. Our subtle flow of constant changes is due to the myriad of mutable energetic influences within and around us, influences such as our thoughts, the food we eat, the people we encounter, the things we do, and the ever-fluctuating conditions we face.

Identical twins may possess the same DNA and may physically appear to be exactly the same. But at the energetic level, their constitutions are worlds different. Just ask the people who know and love them. Their tastes in food, music, and fashion are likely to be very different. Their moods, emotions, thoughts, and behaviors are also likely to be very different. People are often puzzled when I muscle-test them for food allergies and find they are allergic to lemon but not lime, or to Savoy cabbage but not Chinese cabbage.

Because we are accustomed to observing the vicissitudes of life from a purely material, and not an energetic, perspective, we tend to overlook the dynamic, phenomenological variability within and around us. The multiverse may be one, but everything contained within is representative of a separate, complete multiverse.

I recently watched a daytime health-talk show; and, as usual, the "experts" were hyping a super detox formula that was touted as being good for everyone. It truly amazes me how stuck we are on the "one size fits all" mentality. It's likely due to the never-ending marketing pipeline that finds its way directly from the research lab to the media outlets and straight to you. While this mind-shaping hype machine may generate an endless stream of revenue, it continually spews obsolete misinformation. No one nutritional supplement, drug, or food can be good for everyone. When we're dealing with living energy, every living thing has its own separate constitution.

We are all unique and should never allow ourselves to be cattle prodded into the corral of "one size fits all" living. We're all forced to contend with our constitution every day; we're simply not aware of it. Some of us look good in yellow, while others look good in red.

Some of us are drawn to sweet, doughy foods, while others prefer salty foods with a crunch. We're each one of a kind, and we all express individual tendencies that reveal our constitution. Whole Health teaches that the first step to true wholeness is to appreciate the subtle energetic differences between all forms.

Over the years, I have witnessed many examples of constitutional differences among my patients. For example, a woman once told me that she could only correct her hyper-acidity with foods like red meat. Red meat is an acidic food; but, for some, it may actually help absorb excess hydrochloric acid. I recall another woman who insisted that whenever she consumes peppermint tea with any regularity, she tends to lose weight. Then, there was a man who once claimed that he could only regulate his pH (acid/alkaline balance) by consuming a baked potato once a day. We are all microuniverses unto ourselves, together making up a vast macromultiverse. Everywhere you look there are reminders of the multiplicity of constitutions. Recently, the topic of cellular memory theory has provided some interesting perspective regarding the uniqueness of our codes.

As far back as the early 1970s, many heart transplant recipients were noted as having undergone dramatic personality changes that eerily reflected the personality of the donors. Changes in opinion, craving, taste, attitude, and even vocabulary have all been consistently noted in many organ transplant recipients. In his book *The Heart's Code*, neuropsychologist Paul Pearsall tells the story of a three-year-old Arab girl who received the heart of an eight-year-old Jewish boy. One day, the girl mysteriously began asking for a type of rare Jewish candy that neither she nor her family had ever heard of, a candy that had been a favorite of the little boy who was her donor. But the concept of our energetic uniqueness isn't just logical, nor is it complicated. We need only turn to common, day-to-day life scenarios to see our personal energy codes revealed.

Imagine going to a party with a good number of invitees. Over the course of the next several hours you will have the opportunity to meet and chat with many of them. The next morning, as you reflect back on your various party encounters, you will likely recall a blend of great, good, fair, poor, and not-so-great connections. No one personality jibes with all others. Energy must match in order for there to be compatibility. At the subtle energetic level, life is a game of pitch and catch. Some connections spark instantly, some spark a little, and some don't spark at all. And so, it is also true when it comes to the mixing and matching of energies between people, jobs, music, movies, food, vitamins, and medicine. It's all about constitutions.

Whole Health is a healing system that focuses on the profound differentiation of energy and the exchange of energetic influences from one moment to the next. The thing that truly distinguishes this from other healing systems is that it provides the practitioner with tools to decode and master the art of understanding the energetic constitution.

Our energy codes contain and reflect our own, unique information. At an energy level, we all have different quirks, needs, preferences, and tendencies—and we also possess distinctly different spirits, psychologies, and physiologies. Science is beginning to find constitutionality showing up in the most unexpected places.

In June 2012, the Human Microbiome Project published their long-awaited findings, announcing the discovery that we each have our own personal bacterial codes. As it turns out, we all have varying amounts of good and bad bacteria, with a variety of different strains. Moreover, none of our good and bad bacterial populations exhibit the same behaviors. The researchers found that healthy people have "bad" bacteria floating around inside their intestines that live in perfect harmony with their "good" bacteria. They surmised that each bacterial immune system deciphers its own unique way of figuring out how to acclimate itself to the host body. This remarkable research suggests that each of us produce an immunological adaptation reflective of our personal code.

Our constitution codes represent all our most vital information, and in order for us to maximize our balance and wellness, it's essential that we understand the inner workings of our codes. Whole Health asserts that constitution is a vital missing ingredient in our current health care approach. Wellness and disease prevention have become main focuses of medicine, yet we've made no real effort to properly educate patients about their constitutional self. The average patient knows little about good nutrition and even less about their own body, mind, and spirit. When it comes to fixing our broken health care system, patient education in constitution coding might be a good place to start.

In order for each of us to become more willing participants in our own disease prevention, we must become more attuned to our specific individual needs. Without a greater understanding of constitution, there can be no disease prevention. Before we can truly become well as a nation, we must first recover from our chronic "one size fits all" hangover.

CONSTITUTIONAL CODING, PAST AND PRESENT

Our ancestors had no other choice than to be experts on coding. Their survival depended

Every ancient culture established a system whereby they cosmologically linked themselves with the natural world.

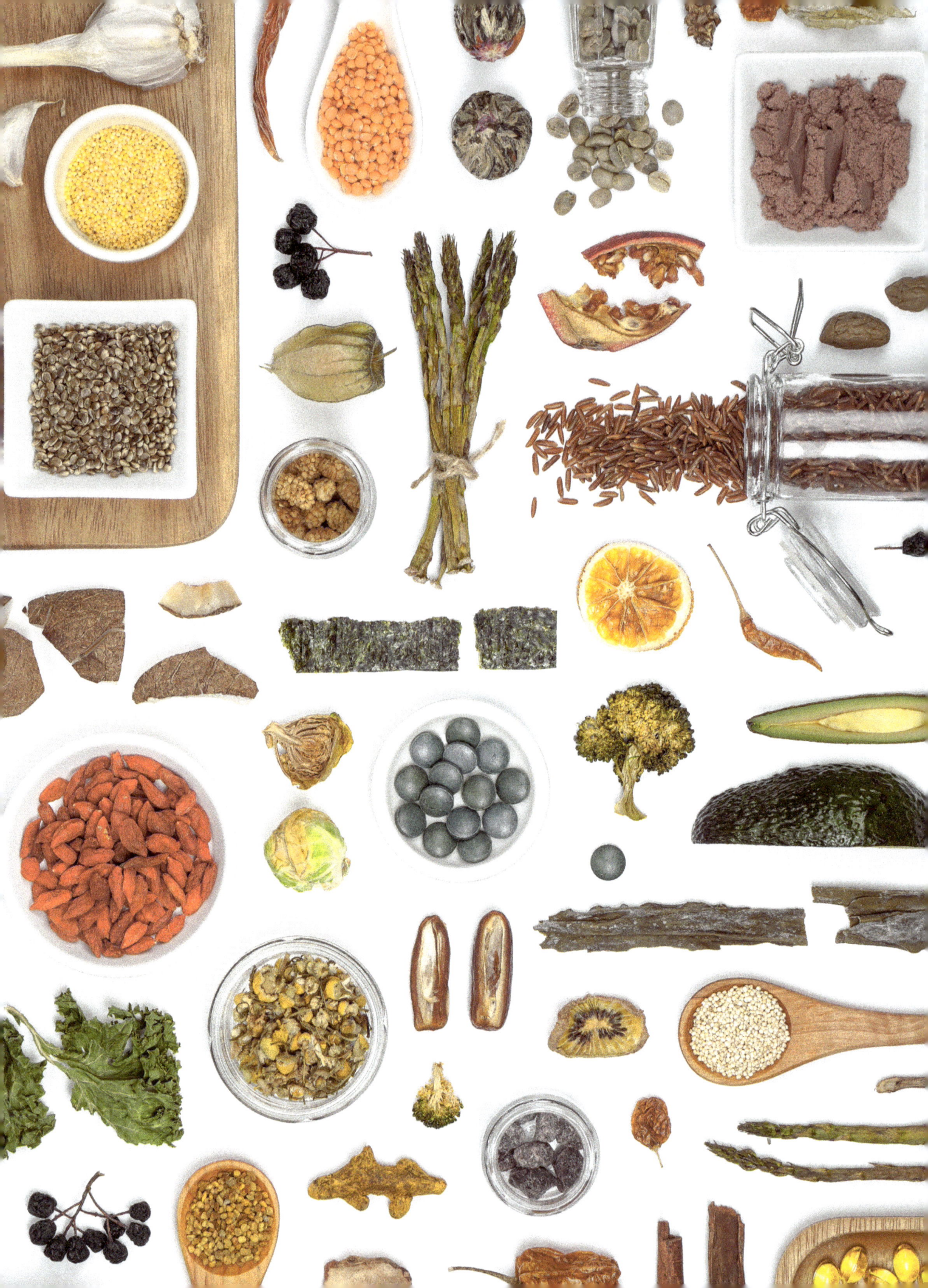

on their mastery of constitutional awareness. They viewed life from a natural cosmological perspective. To them the universe was a vast whole, comprising uniquely different parts, and each part was viewed as a separate microuniverse unto itself. Ancient Egyptian, Greek, Roman, Ayurvedic, and Arabic cultures adopted detailed constitutional systems for their wellbeing and the advancement of their civilizations.

Every ancient culture established a system whereby they cosmologically linked themselves with the natural world in an elemental fashion. That is, they classified different types of human personality types as, say, fire, earth, air, or water. Fire may have been chosen to represent a person with a fiery personality. Air might represent someone inclined to deep, pensive thought. These elemental systems provided them with the means to better understand the uniqueness of each person's constitution, further enabling them to correct energy imbalances that might otherwise result in dis-ease.

Constitution refers to one's general state of health in accordance with the individual's unique tendencies and is believed to be closely related to pathogenesis. It reflects the overall state of body, mind, and spirit. It is a concept related to physiology, psychology, temperament, and behavior. The system employed by the ancient Japanese was called *godai*, and it established the symbols of air, water, ether, fire, and the void to refer to their five different constitutions. The Tibetans established their Bon system of air, water, earth, ether, and fire. The ancient Babylonians differentiated their constitutional types as earth, fire, sky, wind, and sea. The alchemy of medieval and Renaissance Europe was a bit more complex, with an eight-element constitutional concept of air, water, ether, fire, earth, mercury, sulfur, and salt. The ancient Greeks had their four humors, the Hindus their *Tatta* system, and the Buddhists established a constitutional concept called *Mahābhūta.*

The one thing these systems all had in common was their intention to establish a deeper understanding of the energetic uniqueness of each and every person in context with an infinite cosmos of energy. They appreciated that life force defined everything and that everything projected its own personal expression of life force. Moreover, they knew that, when properly deciphered, constitution coding could assist in the maintaining of a balanced life.

According to the system of classical Chinese medicine, there is a detailed constitutional theory called the Five Elements Principle. This system first establishes that there are two primary health-related constitutions: 1) congenital and 2) acquired.

Congenital constitution refers to the general state of health and tendencies a child inherits from his or her parents. Congenital constitution is thought of as the essence (which in today's terms we would call DNA) that a child is born with. Whole Health teaches that the congenital constitution represents our "fixed code," the unique and unalterable aspects of who we are.

Acquired constitution refers to the changing influences that arise from nourishment, lifestyle, and general day-to-day living. The foods we eat, the thoughts we think, the love and lifestyle we cultivate, all play a significant role in balancing the influences of our congenital constitution. Acquired constitution represents what Whole Health calls our "mutable code."

One of the fundamental beliefs of Chinese medicine is that human beings are infinitely intertwined with all of nature. The ancient Chinese classified all of nature into a handful of basic elements.

They mapped out five energetic classifications intended to represent the unique distinctions between everything in nature. They divided the entire multiverse of unseen energy into five separate categories for the purposes of establishing unique distinctions and dynamic contrasts. Here they could

The foods we eat, the thoughts we think, the love and lifestyle we cultivate, all play a significant role in balancing our constitution.

The five classifications of elements pertained to everything in the universe, including you and me.

plainly distinguish the differences and similarities between all things. They understood that to prosper, live, adapt, and survive, they would need to better understand the uniqueness of the energies within the mosaic of life.

To their way of thinking, the universe comprised varying energies that constantly required balancing. This concept was applied directly in their practice of medicine and disease prevention. Balancing your energy would require different foods and medicines than your neighbor would. These constitutional prescriptions would also have to change seasonally, in accordance with the fluidity of nature. What you ate, drank, and took medicinally was constantly changing as the seasons brought forth their respective energetic cycles. There is no one-size-fits-all approach to living—and it is dynamic, not static. They didn't all eat the same wheat, drink the same milk, or take Lipitor forever. Everyone's needs, tendencies, and behaviors were respected and treated in accordance with their ever-changing individual needs.

Each of the five element classifications is associated with a graphic symbol to represent what are believed to be the primary categories of all and everything that exists between heaven and earth. The origins of these five energy distinctions are quite logical, when you think about it.

THE FIVE MANIFESTATIONS OF ENERGY

1. Abundance
2. Excess
3. Balance
4. Deficiency
5. Insufficiency

To the ancients, the universe was a dynamic domain of living change driven by a powerful, unseen life force. They envisioned the circuiting heavens, the changing seasons, the wind, rain, snow, and every living being as an embodiment of one of the five manifestations

of energy. In energy terms, everything either had an abundance, excess, balance, deficiency, or an insufficiency of life force. They understood the vital importance of distinguishing the differences between all energies, so they devised a system with five metaphors that represented the energy differences for all dynamic energies. These became known as the five constitutional elements.

THE FIVE CONSTITUTION CODES (FIXED)

1. **Wood**—abundant energy
2. **Fire**—excess energy
3. **Earth**—balanced energy
4. **Metal**—deficient energy
5. **Water**—insufficient energy

Remember, the five classifications of elements pertained to everything in the universe, including you and me. We all fit somewhere within those five elements.

Within the extended cosmological tapestry of the Five Elements Principle, the ancient Chinese established five metaphors to align with each unique constitutional type. Your first step to Whole Health is deciphering your fixed constitution code. This exercise is Whole Health's attempt to bring each reader to a closer appreciation of their constitutional uniqueness. More advanced study deals specifically with mutable constitution codes and muscle testing. This is where Whole Health truly distinguishes itself as a system that enables its practitioners to tune in to the specific changing needs of every individual. Where the constitution codes break each of us down into five separate types, Whole Health reveals the uniqueness of each and every one of us in a dynamic, ever-changing way. It all begins with constitution.

DECIPHERING YOUR FIXED CONSTITUTION CODE

Deciphering your fixed constitution code is an extremely important step to becoming

Constitution Code Survey

1. Body Type (in early adulthood)

  a. Strong, well-defined
  b. Soft, round
  c. Medium
  d. Medium, lean
  e. Thin, lean

2. Stamina

  a. Good energy, good endurance
  b. High energy, poor endurance
  c. Moderate energy, inconsistent endurance
  d. Low energy, always conserves
  e. Very low energy, physically inactive

3. Health Vulnerability

  a. Liver/digestive
  b. Heart/stress
  c. Spleen/general immune
  d. Lung/allergy
  e. Genito-urinary/hormonal/skeletal

4. Positive Mental Nature (at your best)

  a. Confident, independent
  b. Enthusiastic, exciting
  c. Nurturing, caring
  d. Logical, precise
  e. Cautious, conservative

5. Negative Mental Nature (at your worst)

  a. Obstinate, argumentative
  b. Impulsive, consuming
  c. Meddlesome, manipulative
  d. Obsessive, perfectionistic
  e. Stagnant, withdrawn

6. Positive Emotional Nature (at your best)

  a. Kind, giving
  b. Joyous, optimistic
  c. Compassionate, warm
  d. Courageous, bold
  e. Calm, peaceful

7. Negative Emotional Nature (at your worst)

  a. Angry, impatient
  b. Vengeful, impulsive
  c. Anxious, dysfunctional
  d. Melancholic, depressed
  e. Fearful, disassociated

8. Spiritual Tendency

  a. Agnostic
  b. Mystical
  c. Pantheistic
  d. Orthodox
  e. Unorthodox

9. Your Persona in Your Family Relationships

  a. Performer
  b. Idealist
  c. Peacemaker
  d. Perfectionist
  e. Escapist

10. Your Persona in Your Romantic Relationships

  a. Loyal
  b. Tempestuous
  c. Warm
  d. Detached
  e. Mysterious

11. Sexual Nature

  a. Passionate
  b. Magnetic
  c. Passive
  d. Dispassionate
  e. Erotic

12. Your Persona Under Stress

  a. Persistent
  b. Burned out
  c. Escapist
  d. Intellectual
  e. Avoidant

13. Natural Affinity

  a. To be independent
  b. To feel pleasure
  c. To feel secure
  d. To have order
  e. To be left alone

14. Basic Instinct

  a. To assert
  b. To attract
  c. To nurture
  d. To organize
  e. To continue

15. Life's Purpose

  a. To make an impact
  b. To be loved
  c. To make peace
  d. To systematize
  e. To learn and teach

Total Responses for A, B, C, D & E

Now look at your total for each category. What is the lettered category (A, B, C, D, or E) with the highest total? The letters correspond to the constitutional types below, so if the category with the highest total is A, then you have a Wood constitution. If the highest total is B, then you have a Fire constitution, and so on.

  A. Wood
  B. Fire
  C. Earth
  D. Metal
  E. Water

We all reflect a combination of code tendencies. The goal of this questionnaire is merely to help you identify your Fixed Constitution code.

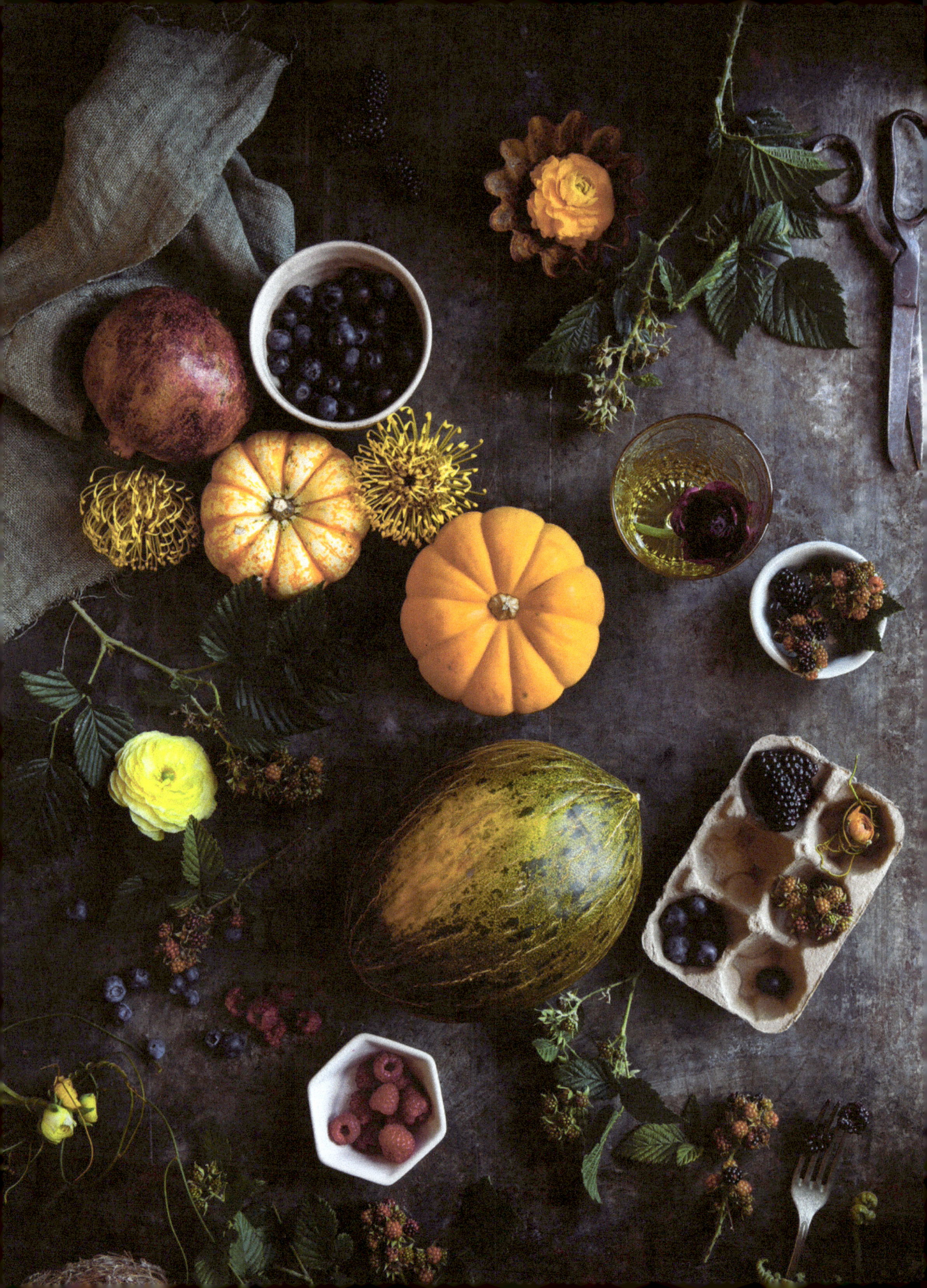

your own self-empowered Whole Health care manager. Remember, we all have fixed constitution codes, which never change, and mutable constitution codes, which are forever changing. The questionnaire on the previous page will help you to determine your fixed constitution code only.

Whole Health has distilled its constitutional decoding process down to fifteen central questions. These fifteen questions represent the keys to unlocking the door to your fixed constitution code. For each category, select the letter corresponding to the response that *best* describes you. **Note:** For questions 1 and 4, please respond with an answer that best describes you during your formative and early adult years, even though you may no longer entirely fit that description.

THE DETAILS OF YOUR FIXED CONSTITUTION CODE

1. WOOD CONSTITUTION

General Constitution: Wood types are impulsive, exciting, and active. They have great strength and conviction and you always know right where they stand. They make honest, true, and loyal friends and partners. Above all else, they are reliable and can be counted on even when the odds are not favorable. Woods must be careful with their tendency to overcommit, however, as they tend to get depleted with all they take on. Woods know no other way but to work until they drop! Wood types should be wary of partnering up with Fire and Metal types, as these are very likely to drain their precious energy. Woods do best with Water types, who are inclined to nurture and replenish them.

Physical (early adult years): Woods are typically defined by a squarely built, well-defined frame. They tend to be of average weight and are rarely overweight. Their complexion is slightly oily, thick, and ruddy. Their hair is dark brown and coarse. Their eyes are usually green, blue-green, or hazel. They tend to have a very strong appetite and are frequently troubled by constipation. Woods have good energy and good endurance with a resting pulse that's quick and vibrant (70–80 beats per minute), but they're very light sleepers. Wood types are a passionate breed, with good sexual stamina.

Mental/Emotional/Spiritual: When at their best mentally, Woods are confident and independent—emotionally they're kind and giving. Spiritually they are often agnostic. Wood types are generally high-performance, loyal, persistent, independent, and assertive. They are Spartans who have a knack for making an impact, but they can be intimidating.

Health Problems: Woods are often bloated, gassy, with a distended abdomen after eating. They tend to have poor dietary discrimination, crave fatty foods, and suffer from acne, dry, burning eyes, muscle cramps, tendonitis, labile hypertension, gallstones, conjunctivitis, hepatitis, glaucoma, Ménière's disease, hormonal imbalances, earaches, impulsive behavior, shingles, mood swings, light sensitivity, blurred vision, cysts, jaundice, myasthenia gravis, gout, and alcoholism.

Balancing Diet: Sour foods are best for wood types, as sour helps their body to gather up energy. The list of strengthening sour foods for Wood types includes nonfermented soy products, barley, Brussels sprouts, cabbage, kohlrabi, leeks, scallions, and most fruits.

Balancing Herbs: Achyranthes, barberry, campsis, chaenomeles, crataegus (hawthorn), elderberry, *Fructus corni* (dogwood), *Fructus mume* (black plum), rose hips from *Rosa laevigatae* (Cherokee rose), the fruit of *Schisandra chinensis*, grapefruit seed extract, hawthorn berry, Oregon grape root, peony, and rose hips.

Whole health reveals the uniqueness of each and every one of us in a dynamic, ever-changing way.

> Wood types are impulsive, exciting, and active. They have great strength and conviction and you always know right where they stand.

Balancing Nutritional Supplements: Homeopathic natrum sulphuricum, hepar sulphuricum, lycopodium, choline, lecithin, and methionine.

2. FIRE CONSTITUTION

General Constitution: Fire types are extremely overactive. They tend to be active even when they are doing nothing. They are distracted, fidgety, and are constantly moving on to the next thing. Fires are intensely passionate, but because they burn so bright, they must be very careful not to burn out. They are inspiring and charismatic, and everything seems to stand still when they enter the room. They have the gift to excite and are themselves very excitable. Fires can vacillate between being magnetic and repellent, as they can be overstimulating at times. There is no middle ground with Fires—Fires are all or nothing. They do best in partnerships with Wood and Earth types but must be careful not to exhaust them. Fires must avoid Water types, as they are inclined to put out their fire.

Physical (early adult years): Fire types tend to have a medium to fuller frame. Their complexion is oily, with a burned brown tint and red cheeks. Their hair tends to be red or brown. Their eyes are often dark brown. They tend to have a constant and strong appetite and their bowels are normal, with occasional constipation when under stress. They have high energy and poor endurance with a resting pulse that's fast (80+ bpm) and irregular. When it comes to sleep, they tend to be insomniacs. Sexually, they are often magnetic and tempestuous. Under duress, they have a tendency to burn out.

Mental/Emotional/Spiritual: When feeling positive, Fires are enthusiastic and exciting as well as joyous and optimistic. When feeling afflicted, they are impulsive, consuming, and often vengeful. Spiritually, they often project a powerful, mystical quality. The Fire type has a tendency toward idealism. They are pleasure-seekers who often get bored very easily. Their natural instinct is to attract. Fires are charismatic, self-concerned, and need constant love and approval.

Health Problems: Fire types often have a tendency toward heartburn. They eat too fast, get hot and sweaty after eating, crave foods constantly, and have red, burning ears. They often suffer from fever blisters on the tongue, varicose veins, rheumatoid arthritis, essential hypertension, Raynaud's disease, heart arrhythmias, hyperthyroidism, Parkinson's disease, multiple sclerosis, hot flashes, mastitis, nervous conditions, fainting spells, hypoglycemia, low blood pressure, acidosis, cerebral palsy, hyperactivity, phlebitis, tremors, day sweats, blood clots, hypochondria, and angina.

Balancing Diet: Fire types are ideally suited energetically for bitter foods. Fires also tend to have an imbalanced excess of energy, which bitter foods release. Examples of balancing bitter foods for Fire types include: shellfish, carrot greens, artichokes, watercress, macadamia nuts, pine nuts, amaranth, quinoa, rye, papaya, olive oil, arugula, asparagus, beet greens, burdock root, daikon radish, dandelion root, kale, romaine lettuce, okra, sprouts, and turnip greens.

Balancing Herbs: Andrographis, barberry root, buplurum root, chaparral, chicory root, chickweed, coptis, echinacea, elecampane, elderflower, gardenia, goldenseal, gotu kola, hawthorn berry, honeysuckle, magnolia flower, milk thistle, myrrh, wild gooseberry, and yellow dock.

Balancing Nutritional Supplements: Omega-3 fish oils, flaxseeds, ubiquinol, GPLC, magnesium asporotate, ace peptides, menaquinone, and serrapeptase.

3. EARTH CONSTITUTION

General Constitution: Earth types are givers, nurturers, and peacemakers. They make the world feel welcomed, cared for, and loved. Regardless of whether they are male or female, Earths all have a mothering quality about them. The problem is they not only give, they give in—they can't seem to say no. Earth types rarely get enough back in return from others, and they tend to ignore their own needs as well. Earth types are not enamored of the latest fashion trends. They're down-home types with a focus on comfort and grounding. They love their homes and are always at their best there. They love raising children and nurturing their mate in every way. They are inclined to intermittent periods of depression and anxiety. If unhappy, they are also inclined to sugar, carbohydrate, and alcohol addictions. They are built for comfort and will seek it to the extreme if stressed. Earths are best suited for partnerships with Fire types and should try to avoid Woods.

Physical (early adult years): Earth types are generally characterized by a broad frame that is typically overweight. Their complexion is smooth, sensitive, well hydrated, and apricot-tinted. They're inclined to have medium brown hair with medium texture, and medium brown eyes. They have a moderate appetite at mealtime and a bigger appetite for dessert. Their elimination tends to be normal to slightly loose under stress. They have moderate energy but erratic endurance. Their pulse tends to be moderate and even (60–70 bpm). They are sound sleepers and have a high requirement for sleep. Sexually, they tend to be somewhat passive, but are very affectionate.

Mental/Emotional/Spiritual: When feeling positive, Earths are supportive and caring. When feeling afflicted, they tend to be meddlesome and manipulative. Emotionally, they are often spiritually pantheistic. They are peacemakers with little stamina for conflict. They have a strong need for security and very much dislike having to adapt to change. Their basic instinct is to be caring and nurturing. Their life's purpose is to heal and make peace. They are mediators who are susceptible to manipulation.

Health Problems: Those with Earth constitutions are prone to chronic phlegmatic conditions. They often suffer from sugar and starch addictions. They tend to suffer from bloat, bloody gums, fever blisters, stiff, aching muscles, fibromyalgia, colitis, gastric ulcers, chronic fatigue, enteritis, anemia, low thyroid, hemorrhoids, diabetes, nausea, parasitosis, athlete's foot, chronic candidiasis, Lyme disease, pancreatic insufficiency, mononucleosis, anal fissures, encephalopathy, Hodgkin's disease, and retroviruses.

Balancing Diet: The diet best suited for the Earth type is a sweet-flavor diet, but not too much, as they are prone to addiction. Also, "sweet" has a much broader meaning than usual here; it refers to sustaining proteins as well as root vegetables and natural sweets. Sweet balances and harmonizes the energy of those with an Earth constitution. Sweet foods include all animal proteins, all beans, beets, carrots, corn, peas, potatoes, sweet potatoes, winter squash, yams, almonds, cashews, pumpkin seeds, sesame seeds, sunflower seeds, walnuts, dairy, barley malt, brown rice syrup, stevia, rice, buckwheat, kamut, millet, oats, spelt, teff, triticale, wheat, and all fruits.

Balancing Herbs: Aloe vera, astragalus, basil, chickweed, cinnamon, codonopsis, cordyceps, fenugreek, licorice, lycium, marshmallow, mullein, red clover, *Schisandra chinensis* fruit, Siberian ginseng, and slippery elm.

Balancing Nutritional Supplements: Propolis, chromium, methyl B12, white chestnut (Bach flower remedy), vitamin A, and gamma E.

Fire types are intensely passionate, but because they burn so bright, they must be very careful not to burn out.

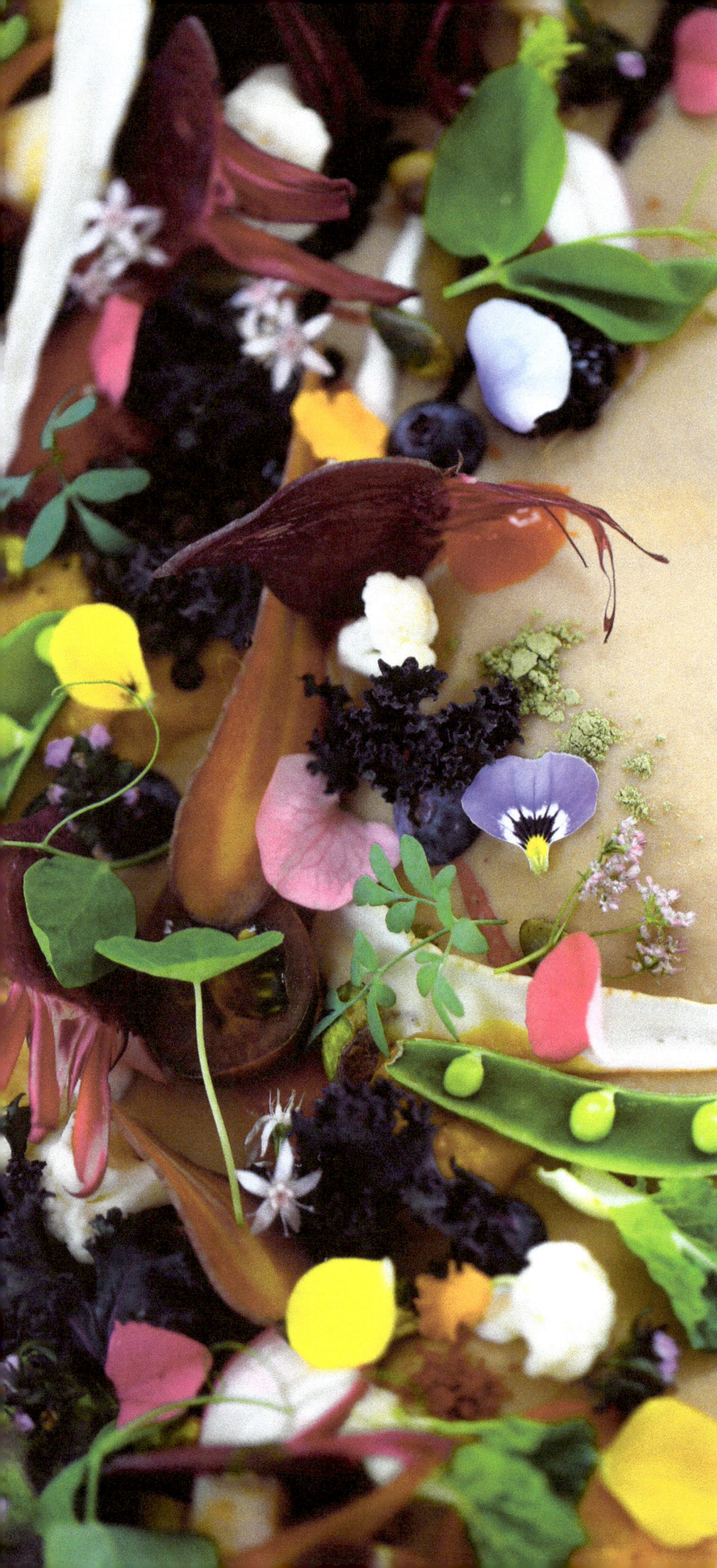

4. METAL CONSTITUTION

General Constitution: Metal types are very exacting people. Everything has to be just right, or else. When it comes to Metal types, cleanliness and order isn't next to godliness, it is godliness! They make great managers and community organizers but can easily draw the ire of those closest to them for completely missing out on the deeper meaning of life. Discerning and mathematical, Metals are the world's greatest problem solvers. They must be very careful, however, not to create problems with their obsessive tendency to solve problems. While they make great providers, they are often criticized for lacking warmth and passion—that is, until they become saddened by the recognition of all the preciousness they've missed out on in life. Then they tend to become so grief-stricken and depressed that they are difficult to tolerate. Metals are wise to avoid commitments with Fire types and are best partnered with the Earth constitution.

Physical (early adult years): The Metal type is generally erect with a medium build. They tend to be ten pounds or more underweight. Their complexion is smooth, sensitive, well hydrated, and with an apricot tint. Their hair is medium blond, platinum, white, or light brown, and of very fine texture. Their eyes are pale blue or light brown. Their appetite is light to moderate. Their bowel movements tend to vacillate between constipation and diarrhea. They have low energy and poor endurance, and their resting pulse is slow and deep (50–60 bpm). They are deep sleepers but have no difficulty waking.

Mental/Emotional/Spiritual: Metals are logical and precise and can be obsessive and ritualistic. When they feel positive, they are courageous and bold. When they feel afflicted, they are melancholic. Spiritually, they tend to be orthodox. Sexually, they are mechanistic and can be dispassionate. They are inclined to be perfectionistic and detached, and are given to overintellectualization. They crave order and don't do well with spontaneity. They love to organize and implement systems. Their perfectionism is their most negative trait. Health Problems: Metal types tend to suffer from bedsores, loss of the sense of smell, asthma, bronchitis, emphysema, sinus infections, allergies, cystic fibrosis, dehydration, nasal polyps, sore throats, strep throat, tracheitis, tonsillitis, pharyngitis, mastoiditis, tuberculosis, chronically inflamed adenoids, appendicitis, Crohn's disease, and irritable bowel syndrome.

Balancing Diet: Metals require pungent (spicy) foods to disperse and balance their energy. These include sardines, bok choy, currants, garlic, ginger, leeks, mustard greens, onions, parsley, parsnips, peppers, radish, scallions, and turnips.

Balancing Herbs: Angelica, anise, arugula, basil, cayenne pepper, chrysanthemum, cinnamon, *Concha ostreae*, coriander, fenugreek, ginger, magnolia flower, mint, mullein, myrrh, os draconis, pepper, skullcap, spearmint, turmeric, and yarrow.

Balancing Nutritional Supplements: gorse (Bach flower remedy), NAC, homeopathic Spongia tosta, vitamin A, and vitamin D.

5.WATER CONSTITUTION

General Constitution: Water types are deep, reflective thinkers. They like to while away the hours reminiscing and contemplating, and are very inclined to meditation and visualization. They make good spiritual students and teachers, mystics, intuitives, and quantum physicists. They are innately inclined to comprehend the deeper meaning of life and are capable of communicating it to others with ease. They may tend to become so reclusive that they become loners. They also have an affinity for losing track of reality, as they become too wrapped up in the world within their mind. Water types are best matched with Metal types but they must try to avoid long-term relationships with Earth types.

Physical (early adult years): Water types have a small, thin frame. They range from average weight to five pounds underweight. Their complexion is cold, clammy, pale, and white. Their eyes are dark blue. They have little or no appetite and tend to contend with frequent diarrhea. They have very low energy and poor endurance. Their resting pulse is very low (40–50 bpm) and shallow. In many cases their sleep is disturbed by frequent urination.

Mental/Emotional/Spiritual: When feeling positive, Waters are cautious, conservative, and have great wisdom. They are also calm and peaceful under ideal circumstances. When feeling afflicted, they are overcome with irrational fears and tend to become disassociated. Spiritually, they are unorthodox. Sexually, they are often drawn to eroticism. They are mysterious escapists who deeply reflect. They like to be left alone, and hate being exposed. They always persevere. They evince a certain genius and they make exceptional teachers. Their archetype is the recluse.

Health Problems: Water types show little interest in food. They often feel faint after eating, crave salt, have dark circles under the eyes, suffer hearing loss, and have chronic lower-back pain. They often suffer from osteoporosis, kidney stones, cystitis, edema, urinary tract infections, lupus, nephritis, sexual infertility/impotence, urinary incontinence, memory loss, insomnia, night sweats, sensory and motor problems, alkalosis, enuresis, syphilis, anorexia, gonorrhea, scoliosis, mercury poisoning, agoraphobia, and bulimia.

Balancing Diet: Salty foods tend to soften, moisten, and balance the kidneys and adrenal glands of the Water type. Among the best

Earth types are givers, nurturers, and peacemakers. They make the world feel welcomed, cared for, and loved.

> Metals are logical and precise and can be obsessive and ritualistic. When they feel positive, they are courageous and bold.

examples of balancing salty foods are sea bass, pinto beans, chestnuts, endive, escarole, Bibb lettuce, Concord grapes, olives, seaweed, sorrel, spinach, and Swiss chard.

Balancing Herbs: Actinolite, cassia, cistanche, clematis, isatis leaf, parsley, red clover, rehmannia, sargassum, scrophularia, kunbu, and natrii sulfas.

Balancing Nutritional Supplements: cranberry capsules, mimulus (Bach flower remedy), homeopathic *Eupatorium purpureum*, zinc gluconate, and raw kidney tablets.

CODE COMPATABILITY

It is important to note that many of the foods and herbs mentioned in the above discussion of "types" generate more than one flavor, and may therefore occupy multiple categories. Each code type energetically affects and is affected by all other code types. Some codes will tend to have a positive influence, while others will tend to have a negative effect on each other. To understand these interconnections, we must perform "code compatibility." When constitutional types are compatibly matched, relationships are very likely to flourish.

Most Compatible Constitutional Matches

1. Woods energize Fires
2. Fires energize Earths
3. Earths energize Metals
4. Metals energize Waters
5. Waters energize Woods

Least Compatible Constitutional Matches

1. Woods deplete Earths
2. Earths deplete Waters
3. Waters deplete Fires
4. Fires deplete Metals
5. Metals deplete Woods

You have initiated the process of identify-

ing your unique energetic identity. In the chapters that follow, Whole Health will teach you to decipher, balance, and adapt to your ever-changing mutable nature, instructing you in how to detail your own constitutional wellness program. You will then be able to create the diet and lifestyle best suited to your specific, ever-changing energy needs.

Excerpted from Whole Health: A Holistic Approach to Healing for the 21st Century.

Mark Mincolla, Ph.D. is a legendary natural health care practitioner who has transformed the lives of many thousands of people over the past 30 years. He has ingeniously integrated ancient Chinese energy techniques with cutting-edge nutritional science in his innovative Electromagnetic Muscle Testing (EMT) system. Mark brings his 30 years of experience as a natural health expert to millions of television viewers and talk radio listeners throughout New England and the nation each week, sharing cutting edge nutrition and natural health information to help followers take control of their lives so that they might better preserve their precious health. He maintains a personal practice in Cohasset, Massachusetts, where he lives. Visit his website: markmincolla.com

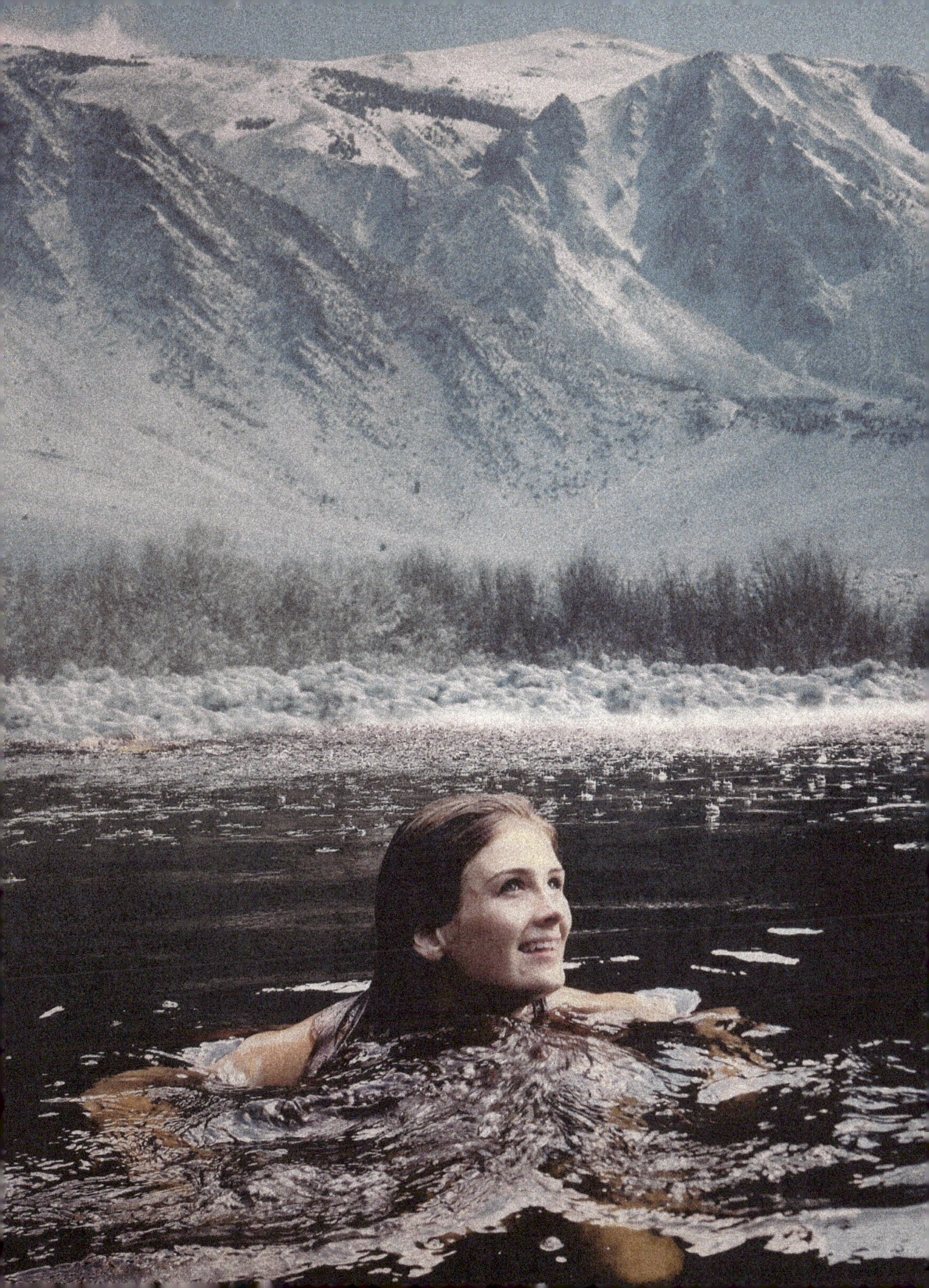

PINE POLLEN: ELIXIR OF THE FOREST

Prized as a powerfully rejuvenating tonic in Asian cultures for thousands of years, Pine Pollen is widely considered to be the most powerful hormone-boosting herb on the planet. But it does far more than just that, boasting an impressive spectrum of exotic, essential nutrients that promote DNA repair, longevity, endurance, and more.

BY JUSTIN FAERMAN

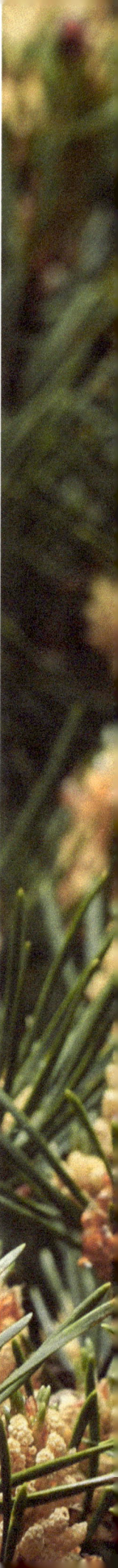

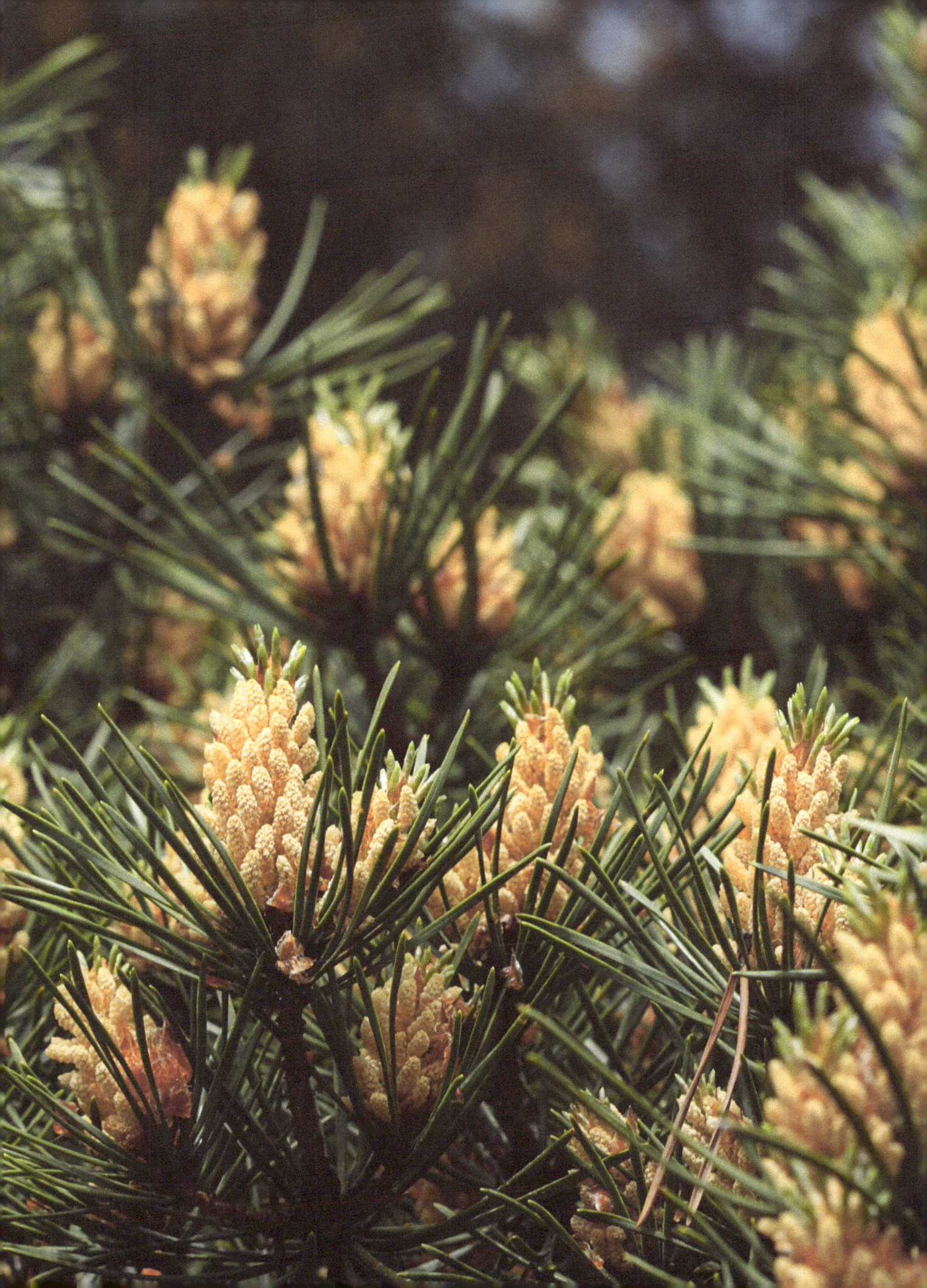

Pine Pollen is considered an adaptogenic herb, meaning that it is one that restores balance to the body.

When one of the most spiritually aware and medically advanced ancient cultures on the planet reveres an herb for thousands of years, there's usually good reason to believe there is something special about it. Such is the case with Pine Pollen, an extremely potent, healing, and nutrient-dense superfood that is proverbially off the radar compared to much less fantastic yet far more popular herbs and plant medicines. With over 200 bioactive nutrients, vitamins, and minerals in high concentrations, Pine Pollen is easily one of the most important herbal medicines on the planet. One of the few substances on earth that has the ability to stimulate measurable testosterone and hormone production, Pine Pollen has been a treasure of Traditional Chinese Medicine and neighboring Asian cultures for the last 3,000 years. Known as a master rejuvenator and adaptogen, the herb has quickly become known to the wider world in recent years.

But just what exactly is so special about it? To understand that, we need to look closely at its origins. Pine Pollen is just that: the pollen of Pine trees. Pollen is a metaphorical seed; and, like all seeds, it contains the fundamental nutrients and essence necessary to grow a towering 100-foot tall Pine tree that can live for hundreds of years. As such, it contains an incredibly wide spectrum and high concentration of unique and rare nutrients that do much the same for the human body as it does for the tree itself: promote rapid growth, rejuvenation, and healing. So much so, in fact, that it is widely considered to be the top natural medicine in the world for such properties.

In Asia, it is traditionally known as a powerful Jing-enhancing herb, which loosely translates to vital essence or life force. Herbs classified as Jing tonics are typically used in cases of weakness, burnout from stress or exhaustion, sexual imbalances (infertility, low libido, erectile dysfunction, etc.), or in any case where there was a need for deep rejuvenation and nourishment. The Daoists believe that we are born with a certain amount of Jing and when it runs out, we die; so, the handful of herbs able to cause the accumulation and restoration of Jing in the body are revered as supreme longevity tonics, of which Pine Pollen is one of the greatest. However, it is also used by health seekers simply looking for an added boost above and beyond their baseline state of health.

Pine Pollen, in addition to all its other medicinal healing properties, is also a nutrient-rich food, containing hundreds of vitamins, minerals, and enzymes that nourish the body at a fundamental level. It's particularly rich in B-vitamins, amino acids—which are the building blocks of protein and heavily influence neurotransmitter production and mood—and Vitamin D3, which is notoriously difficult to get from food, the only other sources being egg yolks and fish, in addition to the sun. Pine Pollen is also rich in more exotic, albeit vitally important, compounds such as nucleic acids (DNA-repairing fragments) and superoxide dismutase, a powerful antioxidant and cell protectant, among many others.

But perhaps the most important and unique property of Pine Pollen is its ability to harmonize and powerfully rejuvenate the endocrine system, which is a rare ability in the plant world. Pine Pollen is nature's most powerful androgen, which essentially translates to a substance that stimulates testosterone production, although other hormones also fall under the title as well. But, if you are a woman, don't let this scare you. The reason Pine Pollen is such a powerful androgen is in large part because it is the only natural source of the "wonder hormone" DHEA, which is the precursor to not just testosterone, but estrogen and progesterone as well. With that being said, all three of these hormones are important for both men and women, just in different proportions, which is why it's important to note that Pine Pollen is considered an adaptogenic herb, meaning that it is one that restores balance to the body by adapting its effects to whatever conditions are present. For this reason, it's safe for both men and women to take, with a few exceptions, which I will discuss later on. But let's focus back in on DHEA and how it affects the body because this is the key to understanding why Pine Pollen is such an incredible herb.

DHEA is the most abundant and important precursor hormone in the human body, meaning that it is the largest raw material your body uses to produce other vital hormones. Imbalances in DHEA levels can and do throw the body's entire hormonal-production cascade out of balance. Furthermore, DHEA production tends to decline as we begin to get older; and many researchers hypothesize that many signs of aging are simply the body reflecting lower levels of DHEA production, which is why Pine Pollen is widely considered to be a longevity-enhancing herb. DHEA production occurs in the adrenal glands, so chronic stress—along with poor diet—tend to affect its production most significantly outside of aging. Low levels of DHEA are associated with immune conditions, low libido, depression, cognitive decline, and accumulation of fat on the body, among other things. Consequently, optimal DHEA levels are associated with improved mood, muscle development, fat loss, increased sex drive, and immunity, as well as a number of other significant benefits that closely mirror the effects of Pine Pollen.

Because the endocrine system, which is highly dependent on DHEA for proper functioning, controls so many different aspects of the body, Pine Pollen is also known in Chinese medicine for affecting many of the major organs of the body as a:

Lung tonic which boosts the immune system and beautifies the skin—two areas that are both controlled by the lung organ system in Chinese Medicine.

Kidney tonic which means that it is highly rejuvenating to the brain, hair, bones and endocrine system, which are controlled by the kidney organ.

Liver tonic which stimulates liver regeneration and regulates bile secretion, which are controlled by the liver organ system.

Heart tonic which increases cardiovascular endurance, raises blood levels of superoxide dismutase, and lowers cholesterol.

Spleen tonic which nourishes the muscles and increases metabolism, which are both governed by the spleen organ system.

Psycho-Spiritual Effects

It is not altogether surprising that pine cones are almost identical in shape to the pineal gland, the master hormone and consciousness-regulating endocrine gland in the body. As such, mystics and occultists throughout history have used the pine cone to symbolically allude the pineal gland. Moreover, recent animal studies have shown that DHEA does significantly boost melatonin production in the pineal gland, which regulates circadian rhythms—our sleep-wake cycles—which are often thrown out of balance by synthetic lights from the various screens we tend to be surrounded with these days.

Furthermore, any plant growing wildly in its natural habitat tends to accumulate Shen, according to Daoist philosophy. Shen roughly translates to the spiritual quality or essence of all things. Due to their massive size and abundance, Pine trees are rarely cultivated, which means that Pine Pollen is almost always wild-harvested and therefore is traditionally a Shen-rich plant. Complementing its positive effects on hormonal levels, which are the master regulators of the expression of consciousness in the body, Pine Pollen tends to make us more connected to nature, our bodies, our essence, and our spirit.

Use and Selection

Pine Pollen is somewhat unique in that the

Pine Pollen is also known in Chinese medicine for affecting many of the major organs of the body.

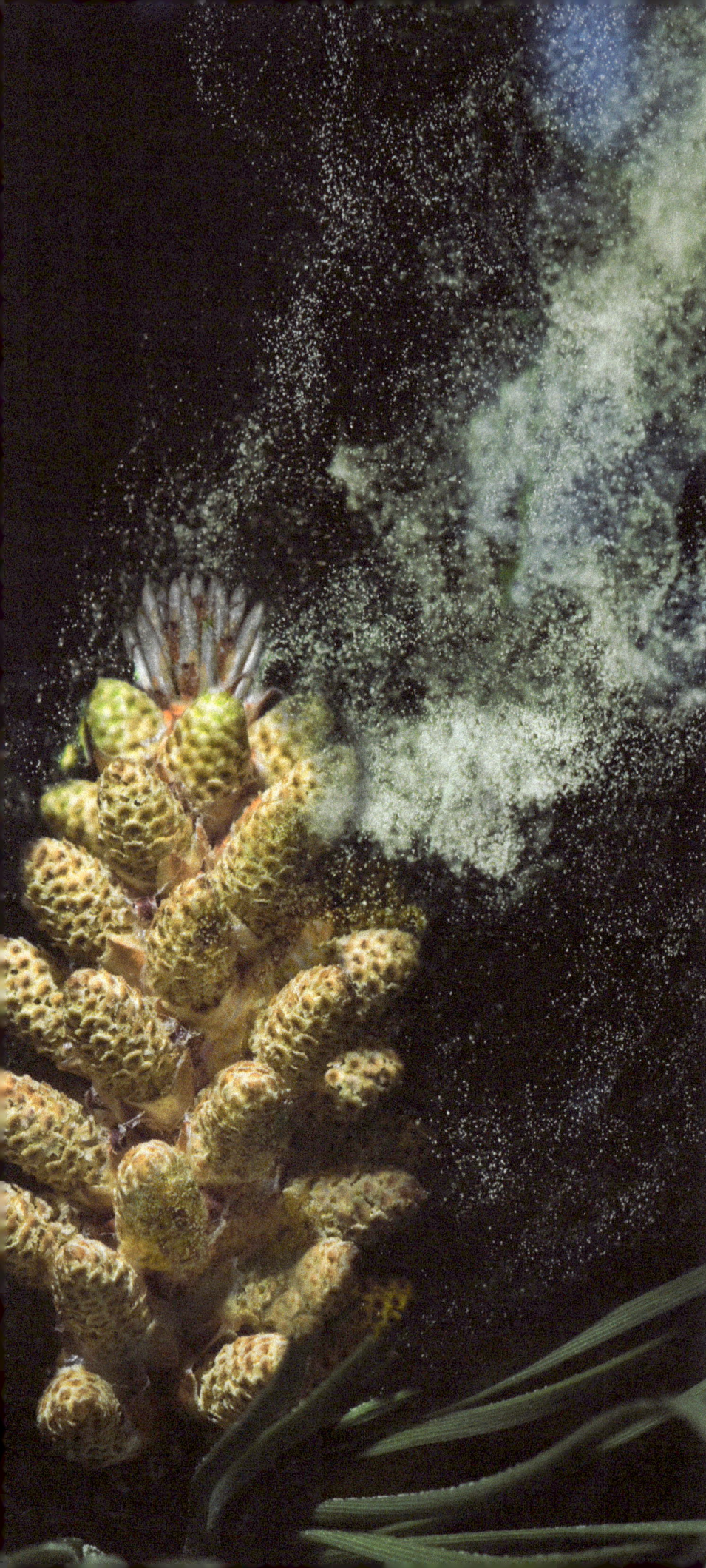

Pine trees from which it is produced grow wildly in many locations across the planet, making it readily available at certain times of the year. As such, many people choose to wild harvest their own from local trees. While that's not practical for most people, the same rules apply to the selection of quality Pine Pollen: look for wildcrafted and wild-harvested products sourced from pollution-free pristine wilderness regions without any fillers or additives.

An interesting thing to note is that Pine Pollen has a thick cell wall to allow it to remain intact through the often-arduous journey of aerial dispersal from the cone buds. As such, it is important to look for cracked cell-wall products, which simply means that the pollen has undergone gentle processing (typically via concentrated air currents) to crack open the tough outer cell wall, which allows for a significantly greater bioavailability of the nutrients within the pollen cells for use by the body. While this is not essential, for example, in the case of wild harvesting yourself, if consuming non-cracked cell wall Pine Pollen, you may need to increase your dosage to compensate for the partial lack of full bioavailability.

It is also important to note that androgens such as testosterone and DHEA can only be absorbed into the bloodstream under the tongue or in the esophagus. They will not survive in the stomach and will be readily excreted by the liver. This means that to get maximum benefit from Pine Pollen its best to mix the raw powder with a tiny bit of water and then hold it under your tongue for a minute or so to allow it to be absorbed buccally.

Although Pine Pollen is safe and beneficial for women in general, because of it's strong androgenic properties, it can influence the sex of an unborn child to male if taken in significant quantities during pregnancy. As such, it is wise to consult with an experienced naturopathic physician, midwife, or herbalist if you are planning on doing so.

And as with any herb, start slow and work

your way up to higher dosages to see how your body reacts, giving it time to adjust accordingly.

Justin Faerman is the co-founder of Conscious Lifestyle Magazine and a sought after coach and teacher, known for his pioneering work in the area of flow. Visit his website: artofflowcoaching.com

Pine Pollen tends to make us more connected to nature, our bodies, our essence, our heart and our spirit.

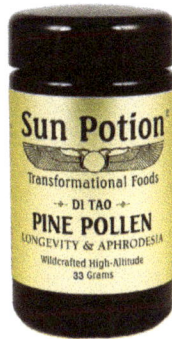

RECOMMENDED PINE POLLEN PRODUCTS

'DI TAO' WILDCRAFTED PINE POLLEN POWDER
Sun Potion

Sun Potion offers a gently cracked cell wall Pine Pollen powder wildcrafted in the 'Di Tao' (authentic source) Yunnan Province of China, where it was first mentioned in ancient Daoist texts.

Learn More
sunpotion.com

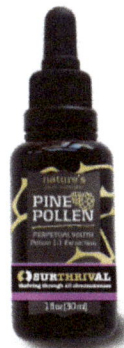

WILD-HARVESTED PINE POLLEN TINCTURE
Surthrival

Surthrival offers a cracked cell wall, wild-harvested Pine Pollen liquid extract for convenient, easy absorption. Packaged in special Miron glass jars, Surthrival uses organic grape alcohol to concentrate the nutrients of Pine Pollen.

Learn More
surthrival.com

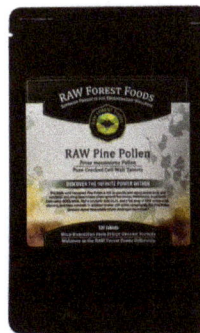

RAW WILD-HARVESTED PINE POLLEN TABLETS
Raw Forest Foods

Raw Forest Foods offers cracked cell wall Pine Pollen tablets wild harvested from robust pine trees at the base of the Himalayan Mountains. Low temperature processing ensures maximum bioavailability of nutrients.

Learn More
rawforestfoods.com

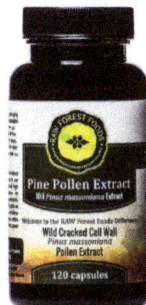

HIGH POTENCY PINE POLLEN CAPSULES
Raw Forest Foods

Raw Forest Foods also offers highly potent 10:1 Pine Pollen extract in convenient vegan capsules for easy ingestion on the go. Wild crafted, cracked cell and low temperature processed to preserve heat sensitive compounds.

Learn More
rawforestfoods.com

A cozy autumn soup using warming spices, savory herbs and seasonal vegetables.

French Lentil Soup with Delicata Squash, Brussels Sprouts & Mushrooms

A cozy autumn soup using warming spices, savory herbs and seasonal vegetables.

BY CLAIRE RAGOZZINO

2 cups cooked french lentils (soak lentils overnight)
1/4 cup extra virgin olive oil
1 onion, diced
4 cloves garlic, minced
4 tbsp ginger, minced
5 tbsp chopped fresh herbs (rosemary, thyme, oregano)
1 medium delicata squash, halved/seeded/cut into ½ in. slices
10 shiitake mushrooms, chopped
5 cups organic vegetable stock
6 cups purified water
1 lemon, juiced
2 tbsp tamari
1 tsp sea salt
6-8 brussels sprouts, trimmed & sliced thinly
1 cup brown beech or enoki mushrooms

Recipe serves 6

Step 1 In a small pot, bring water to a boil and cook the lentils for 10-15 minutes. Careful not to overcook, aim for al dente with a firmer texture. Remove from heat, drain and set aside.

Step 2 In a large soup pot, add the olive oil and onions and cook on medium heat until the onions turn translucent. Add the garlic and ginger, continue to cook, stirring frequently to prevent sticking or burning.

Step 3 Add the herbs and chopped delicata squash. Stir to coat in olive oil, cook for 2-3 minutes before adding the vegetable stock, water and shiitake mushrooms. Cover with a lid and continue to cook for 20-25 minutes, or until the squash is tender.

Step 4 Add the cooked lentils, lemon, tamari and salt. Continue to cook for another 5 minutes. Before serving, throw in the chopped brussels sprouts and remaining mushrooms.

Recipe & Photography by Claire Ragozzino of Vidya Living

Claire Ragozzino *is a certified yoga instructor, plant-based chef, and holistic wellness educator. Blending Ayurvedic principles, plant-based nutrition, and yogic philosophy to cultivate deep inner wisdom for intuitive healing, Claire works with clients around the globe to inspire transformational changes in their health and wellbeing. Whether this means cleansing with the seasons or aligning our daily rhythms in harmony with the moon cycles, her business and blog, Vidya Living, provide a resource for women looking to reconnect with their roots and the ancient wisdom of self-healing through food, breath and conscious movement. Visit her website: vidyaliving.com*

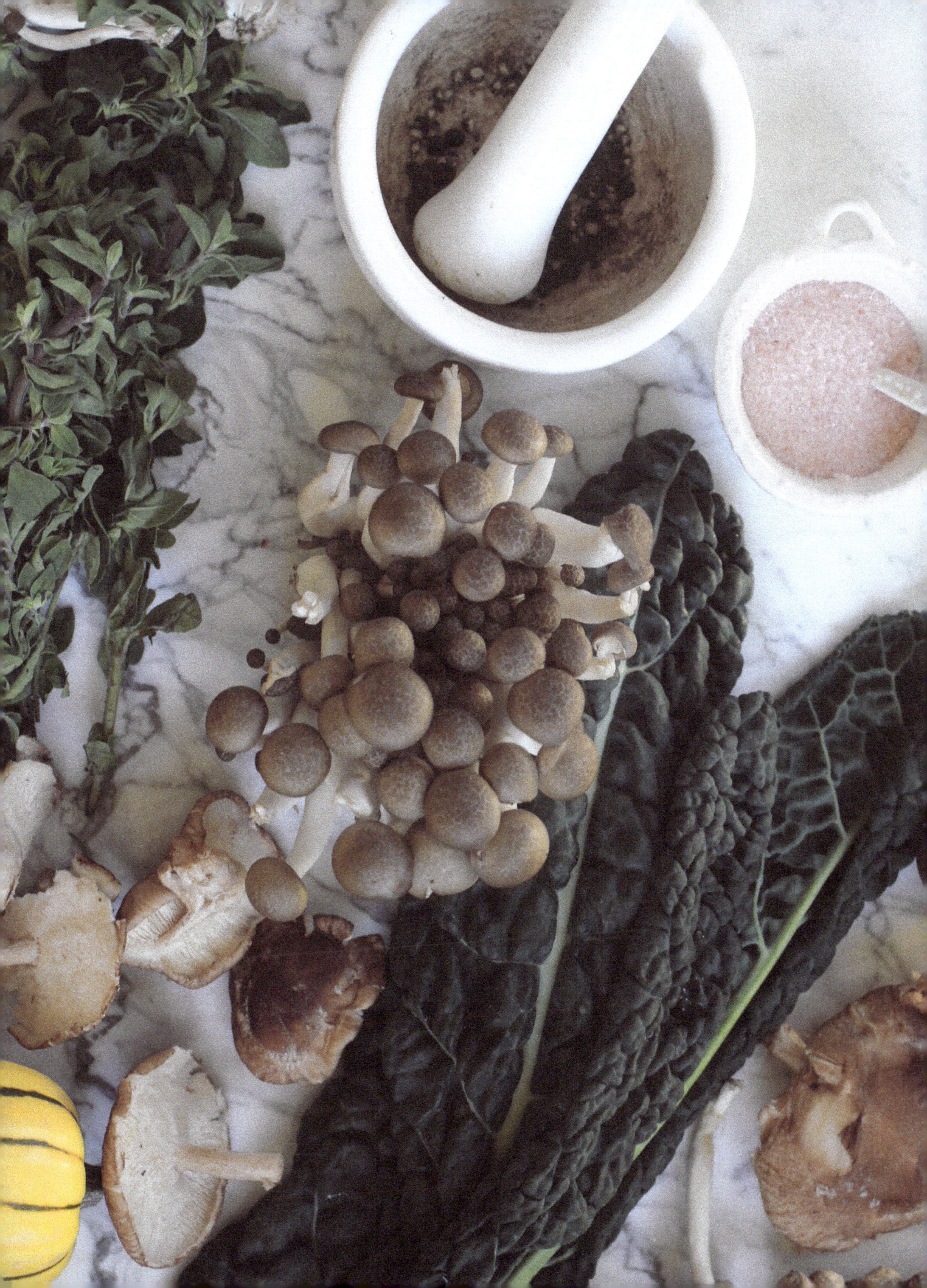

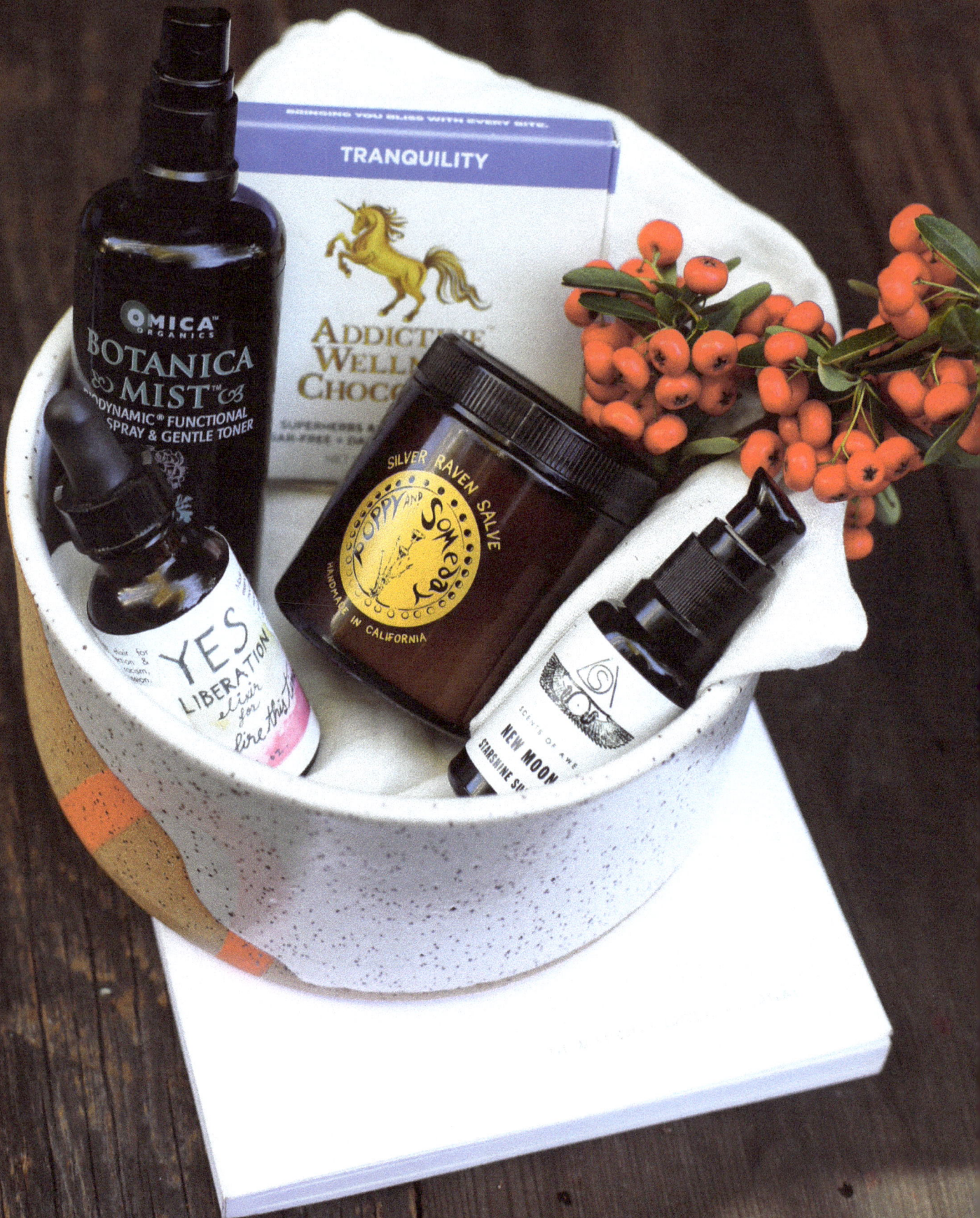

Clean & Conscious Artisan Holiday Gift Guide

Luminary health coach, purity maven & holistic healer Alexa Gray shares her picks for conscious gifts this holiday season and, you know, whenever else…

WORDS & PHOTOS BY ALEXA GRAY

The holidays can get pretty crazy; from buying presents and attending parties to spending time with family, the best gift you can give may just be something that will keep one grounded, centered and feeling great. These heartfelt gifts will connect you to your body, mind and spirit, and are good for both men and women of all ages. All hand crafted by people I admire and have come to know well, they put their soul into their offerings. May you give, receive and find true balance on all levels this holiday season.

Body

New Moon Serum by Scents of Awe - $47 This golden floral liquid is full of anti-inflammatory and nourishing ingredients that illuminate your face to leave you with a shimmering halo. Everything about this is magical and is even made on the new moon.
scentsofawe.com

Raven Salve by Poppy & Someday - $37
This raven salve smells like the holidays and will keep your skin soft and smooth. As the weather changes, oils are a great remedy for any dry or cracked skin, and this blend of organic oils helps expand your lung capacity and ease physical aches and pains.
poppyandsomeday.com

Mind

Tranquility
by Addictive Wellness Chocolate - $8
With all of the holiday desserts we are likely to find ourselves craving sweet things. These tranquility chocolates will surely pacify any soul during a moment of angst or intense craving. Infused with Chinese tonic herbs, full of superfoods, and sugar free, you can indulge and relax knowing you are putting something of real value into your body.
addictivewellness.com

Rose, Geranium & Lavender Biodynamic Hydrosol by Omica Organics - $26
This functional body spray and gentle toner contains ingredients that will calm you from head to toe. When we come into contact with these plants, our nerves begin to relax and breathe easy. With a simple spray you can clear the space and bring about peace.
omicaorganics.com

Spirit

New Moon Journal by Paula Mallis & Danielle Beinstein - $52
New moons are potent times to reflect and set intentions for any upcoming dreams or goals that you're trying to call into your life. This beautiful journal, with original watercolor artwork, combines the ancient wisdom of astrology with practical spiritual guidance to teach you how to align with the new moon and create your own sacred ceremony. Watch as your visions manifest as you progress with the lunar cycle.
newmooncircle.com

YES Liberation Elixir by Dori Landia - $25
Elixirs are a secret way of uplifting oneself and fit nicely in any handbag. This particular one is made with high intentions to help you overcome oppression of any kind and set your heart free.
dorilandia.com

The best gift you can give may just be something that will keep one grounded, centered and feeling great.

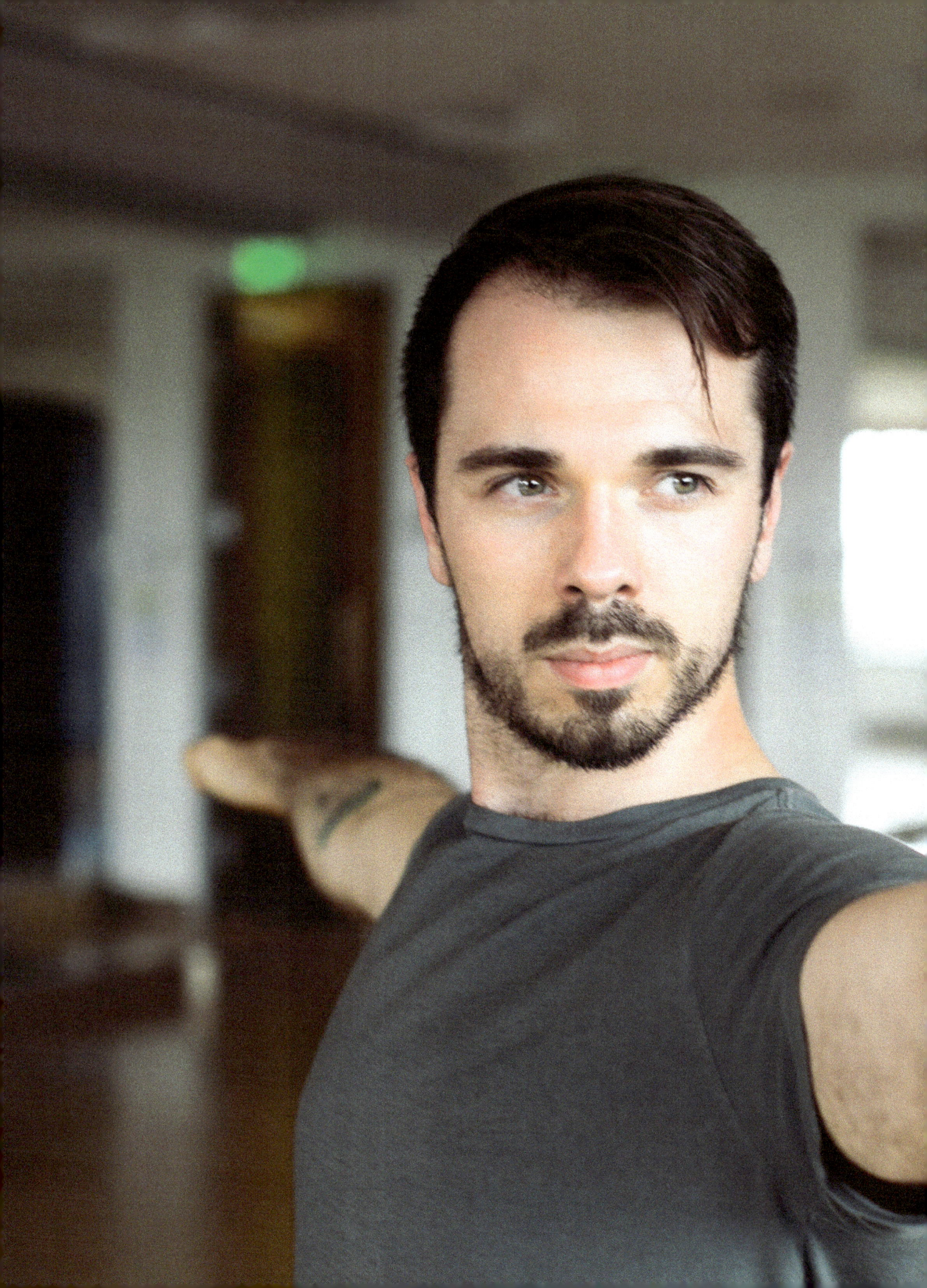

Slowing Down: Yoga to Shift Your Consciousness

Move from doing to being and enjoy the significant positive effects it has in your everyday experience of life

By Matt Cooke

It seems counterintuitive, but what if you slowed down to speed up? To get more done by feeling clarity in the moment. To know exactly how you're feeling, and not have ambiguity about what the next step is. When you slow down to the speed of life, as it unfolds, you move with certainty. As you really experience the moment you are in, fully aware of your environment - the sounds, the smells, and sights—you most importantly slow down your thoughts.

At the end of their yoga practice, many people notice feeling either inwardly focused and relaxed, or feeling energized and ready to conquer the world. Many of us know the power of yoga and movement to improve our posture, increase cardiac output, and improve our immune and nervous systems. During a single session, yoga acutely affects not only our body temperature and physiology, but also helps us slow down our brain and collect our thoughts.

We also know that yoga makes us feel good, but often don't realize how it affects our neurocircuitry. Every posture, including the body language of a pose, creates a certain feeling in the practitioner. When strung together skillfully in a sequence, a teacher can use a class to wake their students up or draw them deeper into themselves. Some poses boost our confidence, power, and strength, while others draw us inward, towards contemplation and deep reflection.

Specifically, the standing postures create a feeling of stimulation and power because many muscle groups must be engaged to safely perform the poses, while in seated and supine (on back) poses tend to lead toward introversion due to the lack of muscular engagement of these poses.

Forward folds are typically passive, using few muscles, with the head facing inward. In forward folds, our physical and metaphysical gaze are turned inward toward introspection. Many forward bends lend themselves to closing the eyes, and slowing down the breath and the nervous system. On a more concrete level, these yoga postures allow us to slow down and still our thought processes. To slow down our mental chatter enough to really examine what is passing through our minds, and if they are old thoughts, to release them, or if they are new insights, to receive them. These postures lead us closer to acceptance and understanding of ourselves and the world around us.

Backbends have a very opposite effect,

The answers were always there inside of you. The question is, can you slow down long enough to feel them?

expanding our awareness to the details of the outside world, stimulating the nervous system, and generally speeding up the breath. These poses work like a natural shot of caffeine to the system. Backbends also typically require much more muscular engagement in the abdomen and diaphragm to keep the spine safe, allowing us to lift and open the heart. If we feel nervous or withdrawn these are great poses to counteract that tendency, and draw our attention outward, toward extraversion.

My favorite postures are the ones that draw us nearer to ourselves. In our technologically rich society, our minds are moving so fast, often eroding our experience of life and our connection to ourselves. And conversely, our bodies are slowing down more than ever before. This weakens our attention to and awareness of our consistent thought patterns, emotions, and habits, not to mention our proprioceptive awareness of our bodies, which leads to dwindling satisfaction of our lives, and results in us missing our personal power.

As we slow down our minds, and stimulate our bodies with the help of our breath, we bring our being more closely into alignment—literally lining up our awareness of our body, mind, and breath. We effectively level out the playing field and draw closer to our primal nature and gut instincts. We begin to listen to our intuition and desires. As a result, we are less stressed, eat less, and follow the natural rhythms of our bodies rather than rely on the conditional power of stimulants and caffeine. Overall, contemplative practices, such as the Creative Warrior Movement process help us to see ourselves with more clarity, creating more decisive actions and leading us to rediscover our personal power!

Creative Warrior Movement

Creative Warrior Movement weaves these two methodologies, with the use of a journal to expound upon your brilliant million-dollar ideas that come up while you are in deep meditative states.

When I studied at the Kripalu Center for Yoga and Health, we were told that what we experience on the yoga mat is like a science laboratory for life off of the yoga mat. A microcosm to express the macrocosm of our lives.

But this can also be reversed to say that you can experience more of your life off of the yoga mat, while you are on the yoga mat. You can begin to feel more clear about the challenge you've been having at work, or in your relationship. You can understand more about your beliefs and fears, and ultimately come to see how whole you truly are. This process on the yoga mat allows you to slow down, step back from your experiences, and get a bird's eye view of your life. To observe all the moving pieces, and be struck with creative insight (our intrinsic body wisdom) about what the right next step is for you. To stop trying to "figure it out," or fester endlessly on the solutions. Instead, you simply allow your body, breath, and mind to do the work.

The answers were always there inside of you. The question is, can you slow down long enough to feel them?

Right now: Slow down, breathe, and ask yourself, "What is my intrinsic wisdom telling me the answers to my challenges are?" Keep a pen and a journal close to you as you explore the poses on the following pages and once you finish, write down any insights or feelings that come up.

Matt Cooke is a neuroscience-based yoga teacher (500 RYT), author, and High Performance Coach who uses movement to unleash high performance for burnt out tech entrepreneurs. Matt studied extensively with Noah Maze and Elena Brower and his work is infused with Kripalu, Iyengar and several coaching methodologies. Having conducted workshops and seminars all over the world, Matt aims to inspire action and embodiment off the yoga mat. To learn more about Matt or get in touch with him, visit: mattcooke.yoga

Bridge Pose
Setu Bandhasana

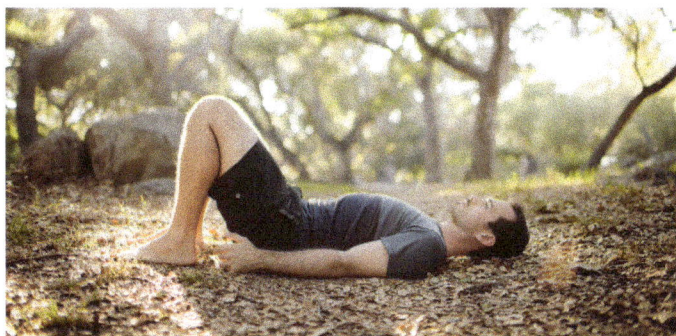

Step 1 Laying on your back, bring your feet to stand right by your sitz bones.

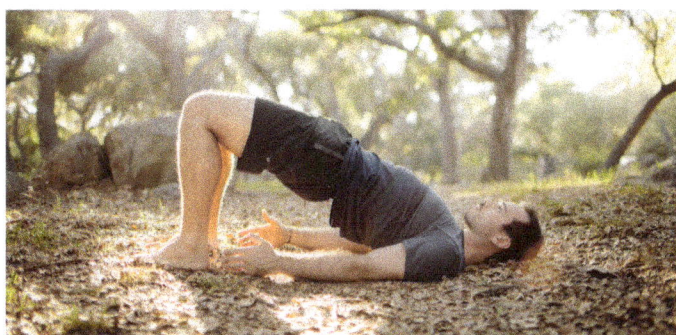

Step 2 Exhale, press through your heels, and lift your hips.

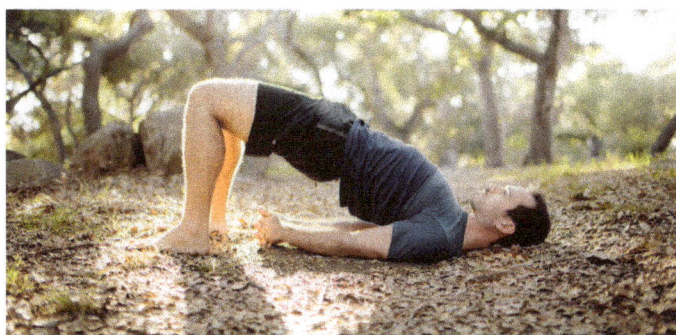

Step 3-5 Wiggle your shoulder blades deep down your back, and clasp your fingertips. Lengthen your tailbone toward the backs of your knees. Stretch the fronts of your thighs. Magnetize your inner thighs together. Press the backs of your shoulders and forearms deep into the floor, to broaden your collarbones.

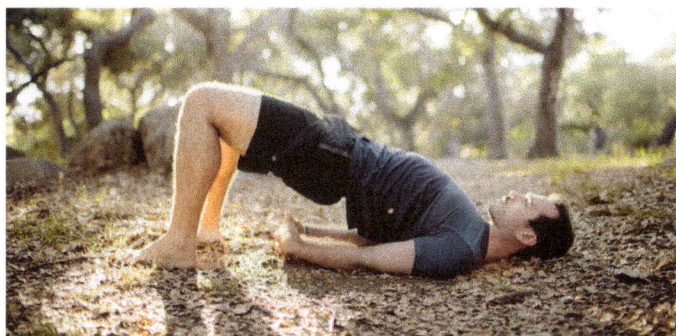

Step 6-7 Lift your chin slightly away from the sternum, and gently lift your sternum back into your chin. Breath in the pose for 30 seconds to 1 minute. Exhale to release. Roll your spine slowly back to the earth.

Wild Thing
Camatkarasana

Step 1-2 Start in Adho Mukha Svanasana (Downward-Facing Dog). Lift your right leg high to the sky. **Note:** *Repeat steps 1-11 in order for each side of the body.*

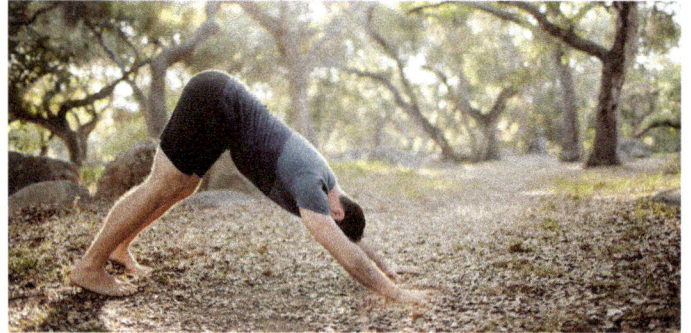

Step 3-4 Bend your knee, and open up your hip. Press your weight into your left hand, and slowly spin onto the outside blade of your left foot. Keep floating your right leg up and over to the left. Externally rotate your upper left shoulder, gliding your left shoulder blade firmly down your back.

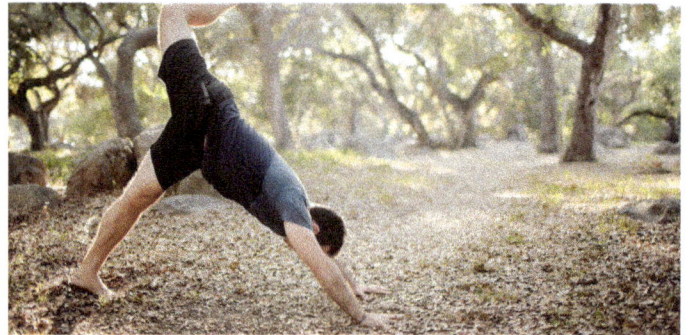

Step 5-8 Keep floating your right leg up and over to the left. Externally rotate your upper left shoulder, gliding your left shoulder blade firmly down your back. Once your foot touches down, in one fluid motion, rotate your torso and hips towards the sky. On inhalation, lift your hips with buoyancy, and lift your heart upward.

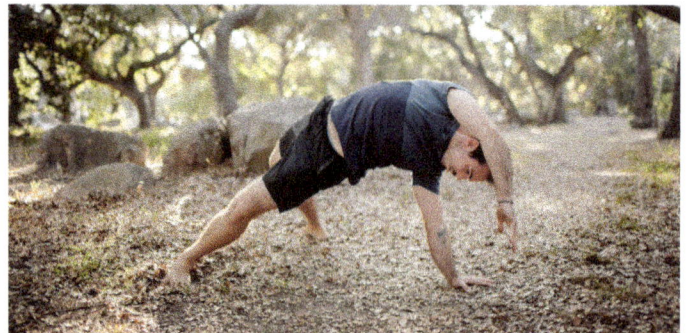

Step 9-11 Let your neck lengthen and bring your gaze in between your eyebrows. Root down through your left hand, clawing your fingertips into the ground, as you continue to lift your hips and torso for 5-10 breaths. **Release:** look back toward your left hand, bring your right hand back, and bring your right hip back up and over, returning back to Down Dog.

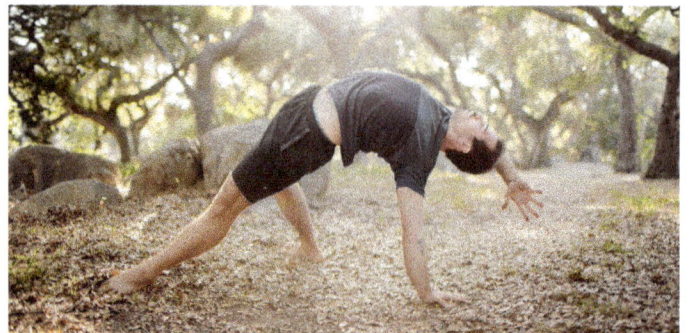

Seated Wide Angle Pose
Upavistha Konasana

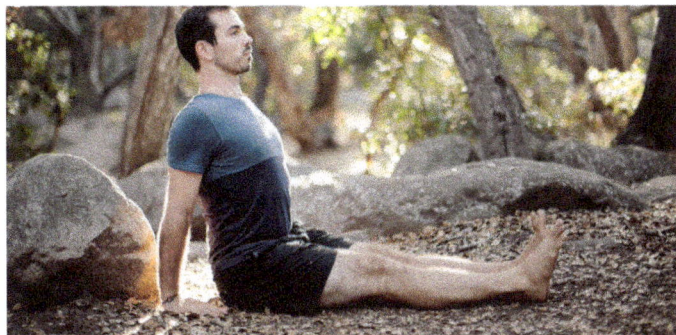

Step 1-2 Sit in Dandasana (Staff Pose). Lean your torso back slightly on your hands and lift and open your legs to a wide angle.

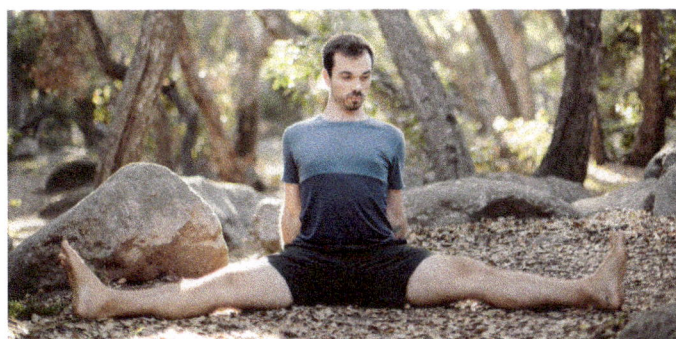

Step 3 Press your hands against the floor and slide your buttocks forward, widening the legs another 10 to 20 degrees. (Raise your hips off the floor with a blanket if you can't sit comfortably.)

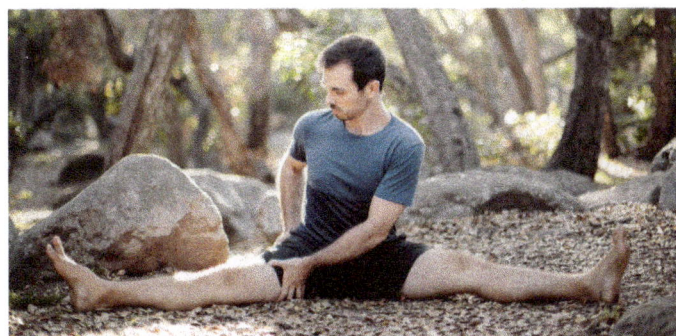

Step 4-6 Take both hands to your right thigh, and rotate the inner thigh down, and outer thigh back; pulling the flesh of your buttocks back with the kneecaps upward, thigh bone down into the earth. Repeat with the other leg. Lift your kneecaps, and press out through the balls of your feet. Walk your hands out, between your legs, keeping your arms extended.

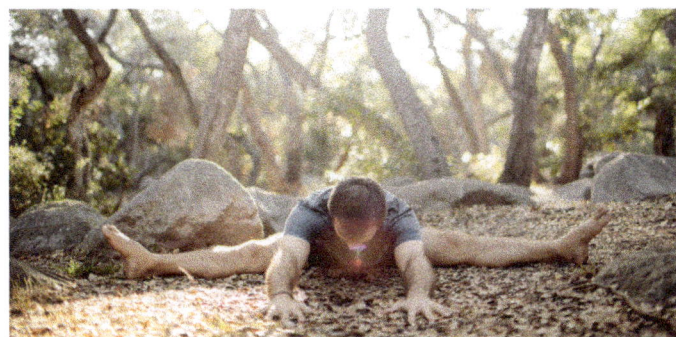

Step 7-10 Hinge at the waist, using your hips to tilt your torso forward, stretching your spine long, as you bow forward. Breathe here for 1-5 min. Turn your attention inward to slowly stretch your lower back. **Modification:** Bend your knees to take any strain off of your lower back and hamstrings. **Release:** Inhale up with long torso bringing the rib cage over your hips and repeat on the other side.

Tortoise Pose
Kurmasana

Step 1 Sit in Dandasana (Staff Pose).

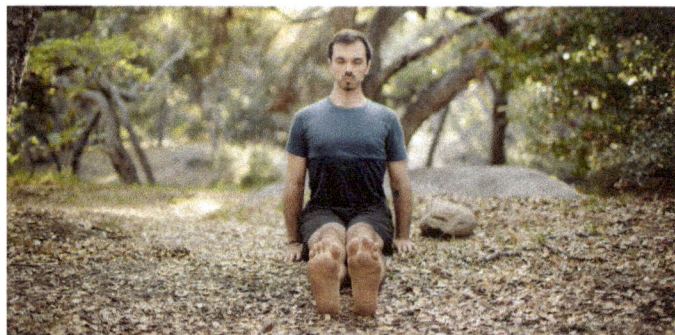

Step 2-4 Walk your heels to the far corners of your mat. Bend your knees to 90 degrees. Draw your sitz bones deep behind you, keeping your kneecaps pointed skyward.

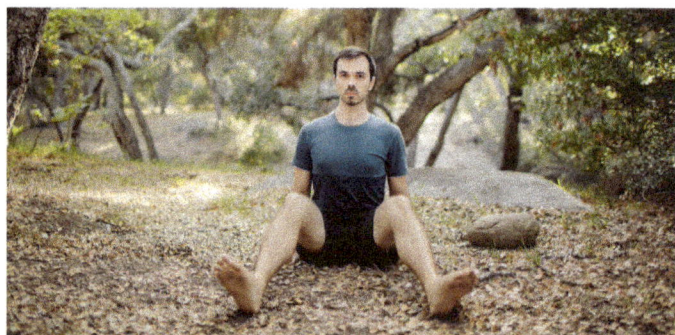

Step 5-7 Bend at your hips and lean forward. With palms facing down, slide one arm at a time, under your thighs and walk your palms away from your legs. Broaden your collarbones, and release your shoulders toward the floor.

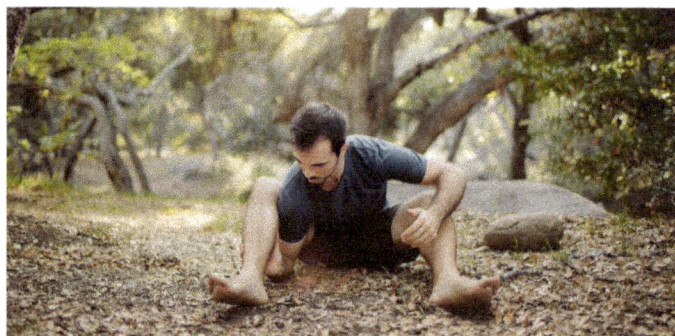

Step 8-10 Work to straighten your legs, lift the kneecaps, & press out through the heels to stretch the legs long. Stretch your arms away from your shoulders. Inhale & stretch your sternum and chin forward. On the exhale, slide your heels farther apart, and reach your forehead forward, toward the floor. Hold for up to 1 min and release by bending your knees and lifting the torso.

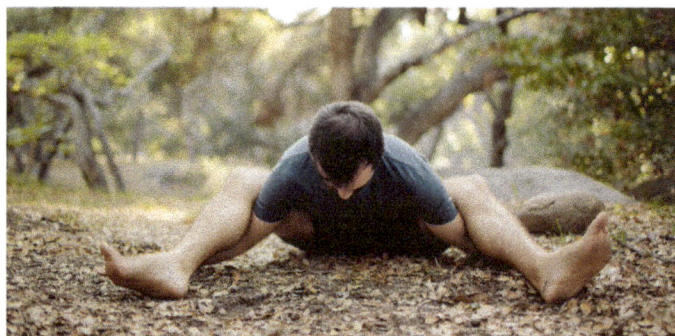

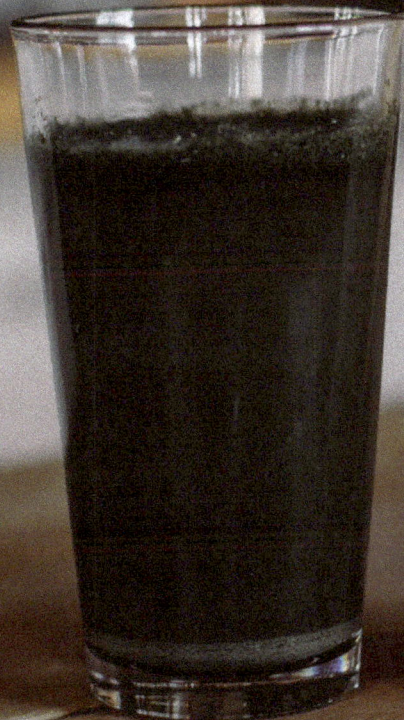

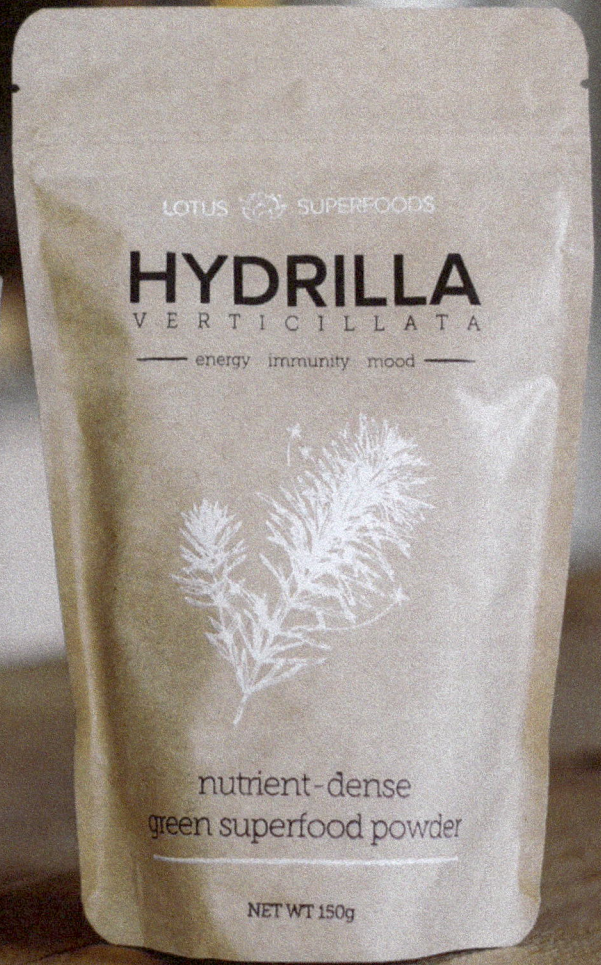

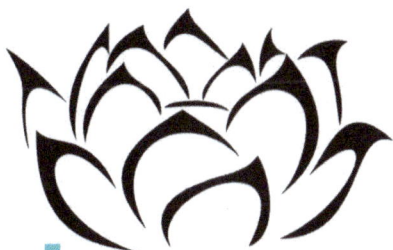

BY DR. RONALD ALEXANDER

The Art of Letting Go

(of what no longer serves you)

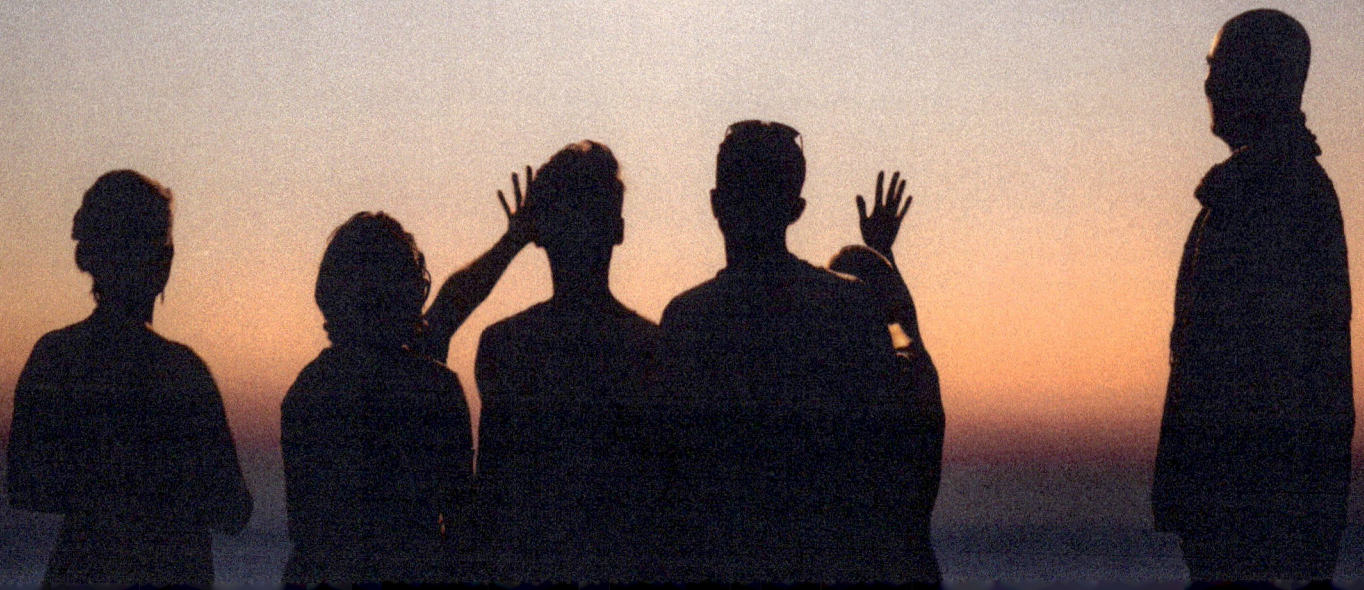

Many people cling to the myth that those who are successful inevitably feel good about themselves and are free from self-doubt and insecurities. Many clients I work with have résumés, personal achievements, and reputations that garner the deepest respect and admiration, yet their negative self-talk is often utterly brutal. Despite their low opinion of themselves, they've managed to fashion lives that many would envy. Yet the disconnection between their inner feelings about themselves and their outer success causes them to hold back from making changes that would lead to far greater fulfillment and equanimity. They'll often remain in a stagnant situation until change is thrust upon them, and then feel overwhelmed by the crisis they face.

One of the greatest obstacles to creative transformation is unwholesome self-judgments, and we all have them. The mind's ability to generate such judgments is very powerful, because it's working off old neural programming that must be rewritten again and again before new, more wholesome thought processes can become habitual. With more wholesome thought patterns in place, crisis becomes less overwhelming, and it's far easier to let go of resistance, tune in to your passions and inner resources, and move forward with confidence.

Becoming more insightful and reflective through mindfulness practice leads to greater awareness of the unwholesome self-judgments produced by your mind. You may be tempted to judge yourself as a bad meditator, or a failure at fixing your low self-esteem, but what you really are is a person making a long and sometimes arduous journey of self-discovery and self-acceptance. Don't hold yourself to unrealistic standards and expect to quickly transform what are often lifelong thinking habits.

The object is to stop assigning meaning to these self-judgments, because once you start to give them weight, they begin to weigh you down. Elaborating on these judgments will cause you to feel constricted by your unwholesome thought processes. Your ability to make breakthroughs, weather crises, and begin living more richly and more authentically will increase once you make a conscious decision to let go of unwholesome self-judgments every time you recognize them.

Discovering & Banishing Hidden, Unwholesome Self-Judgments

Some self-judgments are neutral and don't create strong feelings of anger, joy, sadness, or excitement. They're simply part of your self-definition, and have no emotional baggage attached to them. For one person, the self-judgments "I'm energized by being around other people rather than by being on my own" or "I'm more comfortable in small groups than in larger ones" might not create any emotional response or inspire any disempowering stories about being extroverted or shy. Yet for another person, the very same self-judgments might elicit powerful emotional responses and extensive ruminating if they bubble up to the surface of awareness.

If you're not mindful, you may not notice when the thoughts, feelings, emotions, and sensations connected to a seemingly neutral self-judgment are unwholesome. Often, the rational mind strings together a series of distortions, such as "I'm shy, which is why I'll never find a romantic partner; my shyness makes me unattractive," or "I'm an extrovert. My mother never liked that about me, and it seemed to embarrass my siblings. I probably made a fool of myself many times, being too eager to connect to other people, who look down on me for being emotionally needy." You may not even be fully aware that you're embellishing your self-judgments in an unwholesome way.

Through mindfulness practice and self-inquiry, you can render any unwholesome self-judgments neutral and possibly even wholesome: being "self-centered," focused on resolving inner conflicts, can be seen as negative, but it's very important at times to

When there exists attachment, contemplate impermanence, unsatisfactoriness, and the No Self.
— Buddha

Through mindfulness practice and self-inquiry, you can render any unwholesome self-judgments neutral and even wholesome.

direct your attention to yourself and your needs. For example, if you consider yourself to have the characteristic of "callousness," you might reframe it as the quality of courage. If you see yourself as "weak," consider perceiving yourself as being sensitive to other people's feelings.

You'll never rid yourself of your unwholesome self-judgments and be completely free from the suffering they cause you. However, you can alter their quality, learn from them, and either let them go or transform them so that they no longer block you from a sense of well-being, a feeling of spaciousness, and an openness to new possibilities. Most often, when you let go of your unwholesome self-judgments, you discover aspects of yourself that inspire and vitalize you. You start to have faith that you can live more authentically and richly.

A client of mine came to therapy because she was suffering badly from having been let go from several corporate positions and was now establishing herself as a freelance consultant. She had pervasive feelings of low self-esteem and a continual flow of unwholesome thoughts, such as "I can't earn a good living doing this, because no one will pay me what I was making before" and "Who am I to think I can run my own business?" Despite her obvious ability to procure good jobs, the fact that she had lost so many had shaken her sense of self-worth, even though several of her layoffs were due to corporate restructuring rather than to any failings on her part. Raised in a working-class home, she'd never quite felt she belonged at a major university, where she got her degree, or in a well-paying job with significant responsibilities.

We worked for quite a while to help her uncover and transform, or let go of, her unwholesome self-judgments and accept that there's an upside and a downside to every quality. Over time, she came to see that the perseverance that had led her out of her small town and to the big city, where she thrived, was still a quality she possessed. She was able to acknowledge how her perseverance had served her, as well as how it had held her back: when her companies had restructured or experienced financial difficulties, her unwillingness to recognize the need to look for a new position elsewhere and embrace the fact that change was in the air had resulted in her staying too long and being laid off. By mindfully accepting that she had the quality of "perseverance," which she realized could also take on unwholesome aspects and turn into stubbornness and rigidity, she was able to identify ways in which she might maximize its potential for her and minimize its negative effects. This allowed her to break apart the self-judgments she'd created, experience the flow of her inner resources and strength, and envision being a successful entrepreneur.

You may not realize that your unwholesome judgments of your qualities are holding you back from creative transformation. By tolerating the discomfort of examining your self-judgments and letting unwholesome thoughts, feelings, and sensations arise, you can drain them of their ability to frighten or stifle you. Turning them over to see their flip side allows you to see how you can embrace those qualities, consciously choosing to enhance their positive aspects and limit their negative effects. In a crisis, you can use the wholesome aspects of these qualities to propel you forward out of suffering.

The Most Painful Self-Judgments

Some of our self-judgments are so painful to acknowledge that we prevent our conscious mind from bringing them to the surface of our awareness. We sense that, like the visage of Medusa, they would create so much fear and anguish for us that we'd essentially turn to stone, unable to move out of our suffering. No one wants to face an excruciatingly painful thought such as "I'm a bad parent" or "Important people in my life don't respect me," yet such unwholesome and destructive beliefs about ourselves lie within many of us. Our fear magnifies danger out of all proportion.

By using mindfulness and the art of creative transformation, you can face the truth about yourself and hold on to faith that every one of your qualities can be mined for its beneficial aspects. Your deepest, or core, creativity, the fuel for the greatest breakthroughs in personal growth and transformation, will remain buried deep within your psyche until you acknowledge, examine, and then let go of the unwholesome self-judgments that obscure it.

Avoiding the Pain of Self-Discovery

Mindfulness practice breaks down avoidance behaviors, allowing hidden self-judgments to surface. We're often tempted to minimize their importance, in the vain hope of easing the pain of being aware of our "shortcomings." Often, my clients take pride in what they call their "self-honesty," reporting to me that they simply can't work for anyone else, that they have to be the boss, or that they're by nature aggressive and even offensive in their interactions with others and that can't be changed. Their bravado is an avoidance behavior. Underneath their false, external confidence is a fear that they can't work for anyone else, alter their behavior and take a more effective and nonaggressive approach, or interact with others in a positive, nonoffensive way.

The fear that you can't change may push you into denial and cause you to minimize the consequences of your unproductive behaviors. Whatever you discover about yourself and however painful your discovery, dramatic breakthroughs are always possible. Research on mindfulness meditation shows that qualities we once thought immutable that form temperament and character can actually be altered significantly. By retraining your mind through mindfulness practice, you create new neural networks. If you're aggressive, you can find ways to temper that aspect of yourself, becoming assertive and clear about your boundaries without enter-

ing into a competitive and possibly even hostile mind-set that will sabotage you. Even if you're a lifelong pessimist, you can learn to become more optimistic (Davidson 2000; Siegel 2007).

Working with Your Unwholesome Self-Judgments

As you've learned, the first step in dissolving any unwholesome thought, belief, judgment, emotion, or feeling is simply to watch it arise in your mind. Next, you identify it as wholesome, unwholesome, or neutral, and deal with it accordingly. If it's wholesome, savor it, experiencing it fully and drawing strength and joy from it. If it's unwholesome, come back to it during and after your meditation, and examine the mind patterns that generated it, consciously reshaping those patterns and then reinforcing your new ones through mindfulness practice. This process sounds simple, but you may find that the sensations and emotions accompanying your harsh self-judgments are so painful that you quickly find an excuse to end a session or, if you're not meditating, that you brush away what arises in your consciousness. Yielding to avoidance behaviors blocks the possibility of clearing up any unwholesome self-judgments.

Be assured that even if you were to discover that your unwholesome self-judgment has truth to it, simply making that painful discovery would take you a huge leap forward in your ability to transform that aspect of yourself. Your willingness to acknowledge this painful reality allows you to look at it more objectively and see that there are times when those judgments don't apply—and in fact, they may not apply most of the time. Knowing this can give you further confidence to accept that sometimes you exhibit unwholesome qualities, but you can change that disconcerting reality.

Everyone has qualities worthy of admiration and esteem that serve them well when harnessed. You'll be better able to claim yours and enhance them once you've done the

Some of our self-judgments are so painful to acknowledge that we prevent our conscious mind from bringing them to the surface. awareness.

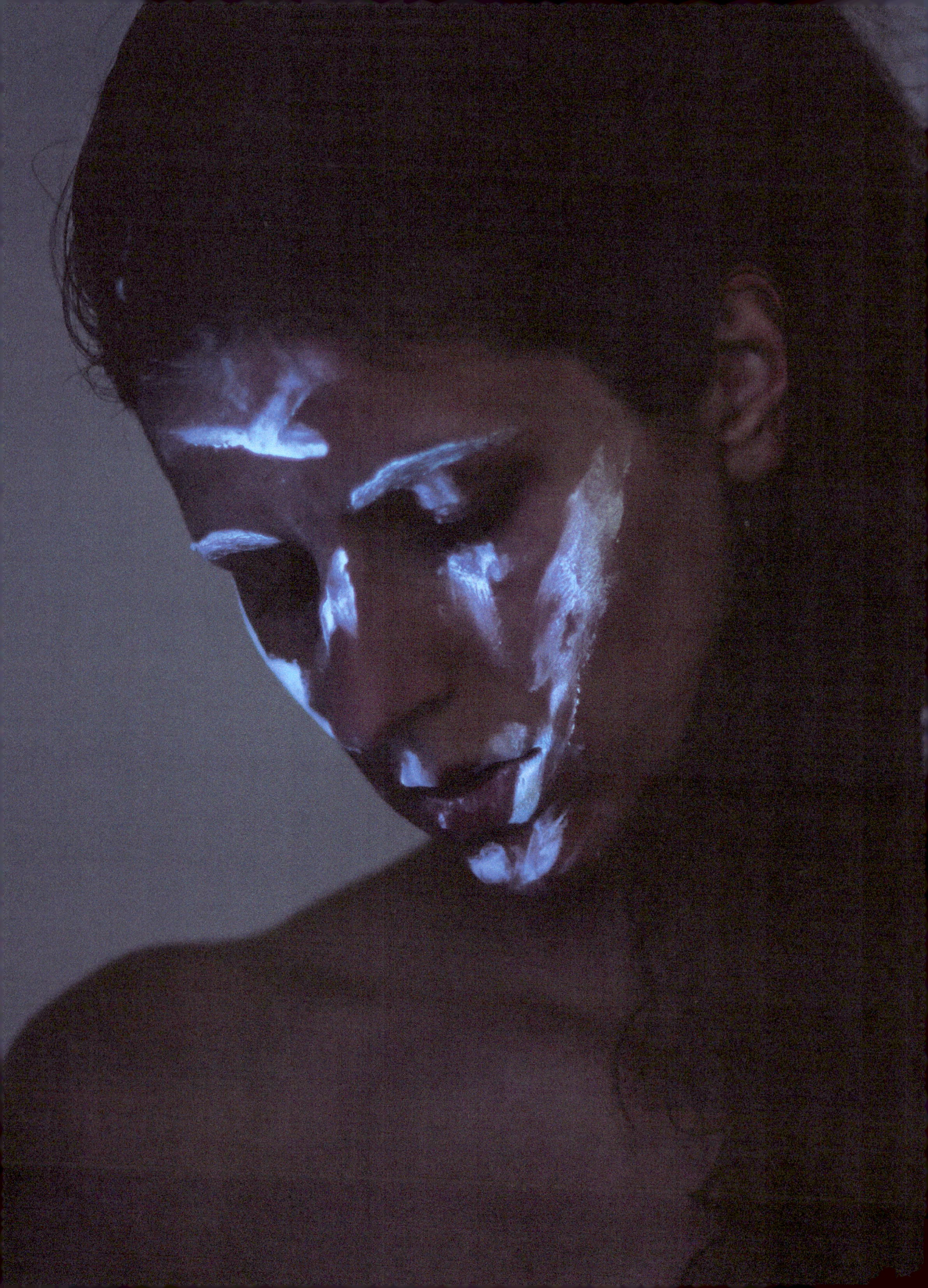

photo: emoji
photocase.com

important work of acknowledging, learning from, and letting go of your unwholesome self-judgments. You may want to begin this process by consciously identifying those unwholesome self-judgments that you know have been plaguing you, using the following mindfulness journal exercise.

Transform Your Unwholesome Self-Judgments

In your mindfulness journal, list what you've always thought of as your negative qualities. Include any criticisms others have made of you that you've been holding onto, whether it's something your siblings and peers used to say about you when you were a child, or what your boss told you in your last annual review. Don't stop to judge whether these judgments are accurate; that step comes next. Simply note what you think of as your flaws.

As your discomfort naturally arises, remain present with it. Recognize that it will soon pass away but for now is a valuable tool for helping you in the process of letting go of your unwholesome self-judgments. Let every painful belief about yourself arise, taking your time to become quiet and mindful, opening yourself up to this flow of awareness from your unconscious mind.

After you've written down all the harsh self-criticisms that have come to you, you may want to group them visually, drawing lines and circles to show connections to their origins, such as when your mother told you, "You move too slowly" or your spouse told you, "You procrastinate all the time." Find the common themes and note them.

Next, ask yourself the following questions about each of these unwholesome self-judgments:

1. Is this true and accurate for me right now?
2. Is it true sometimes? Under what circumstances?
3. Was it true in the past, but no longer?

If your self-judgment is not true and accurate

for you right now, then envision yourself dragging these old beliefs and unwholesome patterns of thought into the trash, as if you were cleaning up your computer's virtual desktop, removing files that are no longer relevant or useful. Be forewarned that even if you make this choice to delete any particular self-judgment, it will probably continue to linger in your unconscious mind, arising again and again, particularly when you slow down and meditate. However, now you'll see it for what it is: an unwholesome, unproductive thought that causes pain and suffering. Be mindful of whenever it reemerges, and set it aside without further examination.

If your self-judgment is true, recognize it as an issue you'll be working with for some time. You can consciously change your tendency to cast that quality in an unwholesome light. Begin to write about ways in which this quality has benefited you or might benefit you in the future. You may even want to use a thesaurus to find words that mean the same thing, because it might shed some light on the various qualities of your self-judgment.

Next, write out an affirmation of the positive aspect of this self-judgment and recite it to yourself several times, while visualizing the positive feeling within your body (this is called an embodiment of the quality), allowing yourself to feel the truth of the statement. For example, see the chart on the previous page.

Allow yourself to experience pride, delight, and comfort as you acknowledge the wholesome aspects of your self-judgment.

As you perform this exercise, you may feel that you're making excuses for yourself, but you're not. The paradox is that you can't acknowledge and drain the destructive power of your unwholesome self-judgments until you're less frightened by them. If you embrace your forthrightness and strength, and practice mindfulness, you'll notice when you're tempted to respond to someone with cruelty and sarcasm, and you'll instantly remember that you want to let go of that old

The first step in dissolving any unwholesome thought, belief, judgment, emotion, or feeling is simply to watch it arise in your mind.

Transforming Self-Judgment

1

Unwholesome Self-Judgment
Disorganized

Wholesome Aspect
Creative, not contained by rigid structures

Affirmation
"I embrace my creativity and fluidity."

2

Unwholesome Self-Judgment
Sarcastic, cruel

Wholesome Aspect
Willing to defend myself and tell it like it is, honest, clever with words

Affirmation
"I am clever, forthright, and strong."

3

Unwholesome Self-Judgment
Unworthy

Wholesome Aspect
Worthiness, deserving, actualized

Affirmation
"I am worthwhile, I have substance, and I feel full and solid within."

4

Unwholesome Self-Judgment
Self-critical

Wholesome Aspect
Admiration and confirmation

Affirmation
"I fill myself up with compassion and acceptance, and I affirm myself."

5

Unwholesome Self-Judgment
Desire

Wholesome Aspect
I have passion and fire

Affirmation
"I admire others and appreciate everybody's uniqueness, and I aspire to greatness."

6

Unwholesome Self-Judgment
Envy

Wholesome Aspect
I expect more of myself

Affirmation
"I am satisfied with contentment and equanimity."

7

Unwholesome Self-Judgment
Sad

Wholesome Aspect
I am wide open with deep feelings.

Affirmation
"My sadness breaks my heart open to feel compassion and grief."

behavior pattern. You'll begin to enhance the new neural network in your brain that fosters an awareness of your forthrightness and strength, and open up to your compassion and kindness. You'll stop feeling guilty and denying your tendency to be sarcastic, because you'll be compassionate toward yourself. Your compassion toward others will dissolve your desire to issue a cutting remark. Then, when your spouse or coworker makes a comment that you disagree with or that makes you uncomfortable, you'll be able to

consciously choose a new, more wholesome and productive way of responding, changing the tenor of your relationship with them and fostering better relationships.

If your unwholesome self-judgments are particularly difficult to let go of, take heart in knowing that the approach of mindfulness-based cognitive therapy has been shown to be very effective with the most persistent unwholesome self-judgments that cause depressive thoughts and repeated relapses of clinical depression. In fact, this dual approach

is more effective than most other psycho-therapeutic approaches, including the use of antidepressant medication alone (Segal, Williams, and Teasdale 2002, 24–25). You don't have to allow old behavior patterns to sabotage your relationships with others or cause you to avoid addressing problems in a situation, setting yourself up for crisis.

Mulching Your Unwholesome Self-Judgments

Mulching has become something of a lost art.

A good gardener knows that organic waste material can be placed in a mulch pile, where bacteria will break it down and turn it into fertilizer for growing something new. You can do the same with your unwholesome self-judgments, transforming them into the nutrients that will nourish your new self.

You transform your self-judgments by learning from them and discovering what they have to offer you. Whether it's an old unwholesome self-judgment that pops up here and there even though you've consciously rejected it, or one that you've only recently become aware of that's true and accurate today, the process is the same. Rather than ignore the moldy raspberries in the refrigerator or the dying leaves on your rosebush, you remove them and use them for mulch to enrich your life and allow you to grow something new. Like the painter or songwriter who mines the pain of her past to create a masterful work of art, or the former drug user who uses what he knows about addiction to help others address their own drug use, you may end up reinventing your life. Then again, you may simply discover that examining your thoughts and feelings about yourself yields insights into what you most want in your life, and how you might go about achieving it. Mulching allows you to turn any crisis into an opportunity and to use your unwholesome feelings and thoughts as fodder for personal exploration.

A client of mine, Alan, was embarrassed at a party after the conversation turned to a subject he felt he couldn't speak to, because he didn't have the education that the other party guests had. He explored with me his unwholesome self-judgment that was causing his pain that evening: "I'm unsophisticated." We talked about how he defined "unsophisticated" and whether or not it truly mattered to him if he couldn't easily contribute to the kinds of conversations he'd often felt left out of when talking to more-educated people. He rejected the idea that to be educated is to have certain tastes and interests, but said he still felt "unsophisticated."

I asked him, "Are you curious about whether there's any upside to being 'unsophisticated'?" Examining that idea, Alan decided that being "unsophisticated" had allowed him to focus on developing knowledge in areas he felt were more important than the topics his friends discussed. It allowed him to experience what Buddhists call "beginner's mind," a state of openness to learning that allows us to connect to our core self and its resources instead of closing down our creativity and believing we've learned all that we really need to learn.

Alan also realized that he did want to know more about one of the subjects a guest had raised, but had been feeling overextended and unable to devote time to educating himself in that area. He felt his guilt and frustration, and then let it go. He acknowledged that it wasn't an important enough topic to justify his view of himself as "unsophisticated" or inferior for not knowing more about it, and made a conscious decision to devote a specific block of time to taking a short course on the subject. The feeling of inadequacy that underlay this unwholesome self-judgment was part of his big story, the overarching narrative that he unknowingly created in childhood when he struggled in school and was told by his parents and teachers that he wasn't "college material." He recognized that the feeling and self-judgment was simply detritus churned up by his mind.

After consciously deciding that he really didn't care about "sophistication," Alan struggled with letting go of the old belief and putting into place a new view of himself. Over time, he was able to use mindstrength to install in his mind this new view and to overwrite "I'm unsophisticated" whenever it came into his awareness. In this way, his self-judgment actually supported his self-development the way nutrients in soil enhance a plant's growth. He broke down the self-judgment, extricated and used what was of value, and then discarded the rest.

> Become quiet and mindful, opening yourself up to this flow of awareness from your unconscious mind.

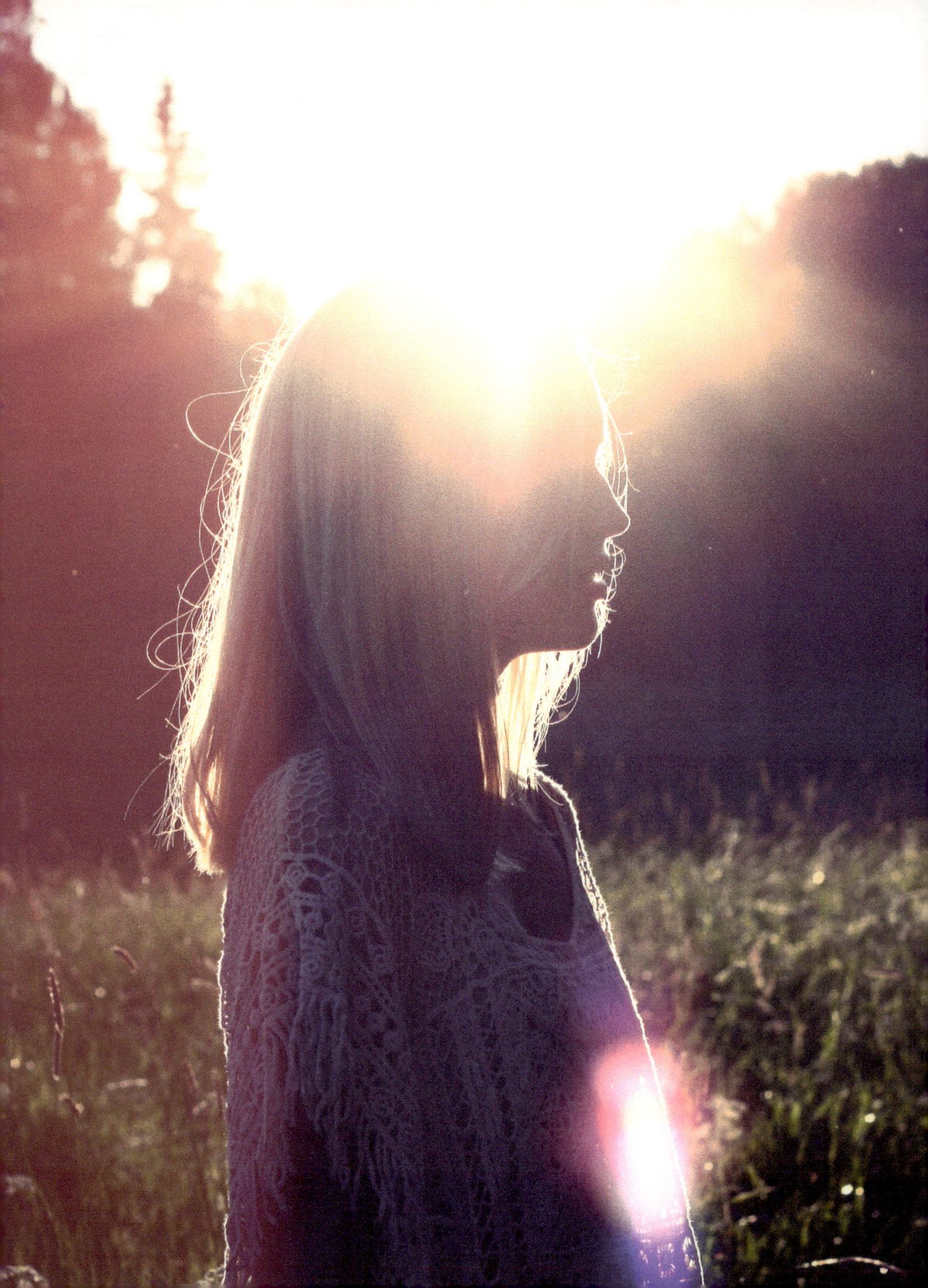

photo: julia caesar

When you mulch your self-criticisms, you bring yourself into balance as you acknowledge the wholesome aspects of a quality as well as its unwholesome aspects, instead of being drawn in to the distorted belief that this quality exists inside you only in its unwholesome aspect. You discover the value in that quality and use it as nourishment while you let go of your negative judgment of it. For example, by discarding a label like "helicopter parent," and validating your close monitoring and careful guidance of your child, you help her move past the boundaries of her comfort zone and possibly discover that she has strength and coping abilities that neither you nor she had recognized. You acknowledge the unwholesome aspect of "hovering" and consciously choose to cease that behavior whenever you notice it, because you recognize that it doesn't serve you or your child. This discernment process allows you to transform an unwholesome self-judgment into a useful observation of how you operate, an insight that will help you embrace change.

In a crisis, it's difficult enough to tolerate the pain of loss without adding in the pain of acknowledging your qualities that sometimes manifest in an unwholesome way. With mindstrength, you'll be able to handle this extra layer of suffering. If you trust in the art of creative transformation, you'll feel reassured that this layer will dissipate very soon as a result of your engaging in this mulching process. You'll recognize that you're fertilizing and enriching the soil beneath you, allowing yourself to grow a new garden of self. You'll develop the strength to withstand even the most devastating crisis, because you'll know that in time you'll bring forth something new that's organic and rich.

The Courage to Uncover Your Unwholesome Self-Judgments

In therapy, I can work with a client to examine the smallest of decisions that people tend to overlook in the course of a day. Cultivate mindfulness, and the witnessing self will arise unexpectedly as you go about your activities, alerting you to your entire mind-body awareness, including your discomfort. You may experience mindfulness as a flashlight that spotlights awareness of your conscience, or as a little voice whispering to you. When you're engaged in an angry confrontation, you might suddenly realize, "I don't like this; it's not good for me or the other person, and I need to stop." As you talk to your friend about her recent success, you'll notice as your envy mounts, and you'll think, "I'm really uncomfortable with what she's telling me. I need to explore the reason."

You may choose to take the time out to examine your self-judgments immediately, or you may come back to them later, when you're alone or with someone on your wisdom council of support.

Wisdom Council of Support

Ask for help from a therapist, mentor, or wise partner from your wisdom council of support, someone who can help you to honestly examine your unwholesome self-judgments.

The following mindfulness journal exercise is one you can also engage in mentally any time you notice that you're engaging in self-criticism. Until you develop greater mindstrength, you'll likely silence the witnessing mind that calls attention to your discomfort, and need to explore the incident later, in detail, to discover what unwholesome self-judgments are causing your suffering. As you continue your mindfulness practice, however, you'll be able to stop in the moment and quickly go through these five steps, easing your discomfort and letting go of the unwholesome self-judgments that are part of your big story.

Discard an Unwholesome Self-Judgment

These are the steps to discarding an unwholesome self-judgment that you know is of no use to you and that causes you anguish. Use your mindfulness journal to work through

You transform your self-judgments by learning from them and discovering what they have to offer you.

When you mulch your self-criticisms, you bring yourself into balance as you acknowledge the wholesome aspects.

each step.

1. Identity and label the judgment. Give it a simple name or theme, such as "inadequate provider," "insincere," or "people pleaser."

2. Discover the quality of the judgment. Ask yourself, "What is this self-judgment causing me to think or feel about myself in this moment?" Does it make you feel ashamed, angry, or guilty, for example? Notice whether the feeling is wholesome and supportive of your well-being, or unwholesome, making it difficult for you to enter a state of spaciousness, openness, and trust.

3. Find a remedy for the unwholesome thought or feeling. Ask yourself, "Would I like to think or feel something different? What thought or feeling could I generate to shift myself out of this unwholesome state?"

4. Formulate a new thought, image, or feeling, and begin to hold on to it firmly. Experience it in your mind's eye and in your body. Feel a wholesome sensation, such as relaxation, excitement, or expansiveness.

5. Assess whether you've shifted. Ask yourself, "Have I shifted out of the feeling, state, or thought that was unwholesome and let go of my negative self-judgment?" If you have, then enjoy the new sensations, feelings, and thoughts you've generated as a remedy. If not, go back and repeat steps 1 through 4.

The following Fertile Ground meditation uses guided imagery to help you mulch your self-judgments. It's a good idea to use this in conjunction with the previous mindfulness journal exercise, because it supports your conscious decision to stop engaging in self-criticism, and actually reprograms the brain by creating a new, more wholesome experience—albeit one that's happening in your mind.

Fertile Ground Meditation

As you sit, breathing in and out with long, slow breaths, focus your attention on your mind's eye, the space between your eyebrows that's also known as the "third eye" or "spiritual center." Bring mindful awareness to each and every negative, self-judgmental thought that arises, and watch for a theme to reveal itself (such as "bad person," "insincere," "inadequate," and so on).

Notice whether an unpleasant or uncomfortable feeling or sensation accompanies these unwholesome self-judgments. In your mind's eye, surround your self-judgment with a powerful beam of white light (or, if it's a sensation, imagine the white light surrounding the area in your body where you're experiencing it). Focus your mind, controlling this white light as if it were a powerful laser beam. Move the beam and the thought, feeling, or sensation enclosed within its circle of light away from your body and mind and into the earth. Watch as it sinks into the soil, intermingling with the rich, brown earth, which infuses it with nutrients as your laser beam turns into the diffuse, golden light of the sun, expanding outward, enveloping you, and warming the earth.

Bask in this sunlight as you feel roots beginning to extend downward from your feet, reaching into the nourishing earth and stretching outward. Then, drink in the healthy nutrients in that soil, pulling them up through your roots. Enjoy the feeling of strength that you create as you draw in power and nourishment.

Wholesome Memories as Antidotes

Memories can be greatly distorted by strong, painful emotions that caused you to create unwholesome, distorted self-judgments. Returning to the original trauma from the safety of the present, particularly with a supportive therapist at your side, can allow you to look again at how events unfolded, using your logical mind to make sense of what you see with your mind's eye. When immersed in the original experience, you probably overlooked evidence that contradicted your emotional reality. As I mentioned before, when the children in my first-grade class laughed at my slurred speech that awful day when I was forced to speak in front of them, my emotional reality was that everyone laughed and no one showed support. In reality, such extremes are unlikely. In returning to such a memory, you might remember that one child shushed the others or that the teacher scolded those who were laughing. As you recall this evidence that the incident wasn't entirely negative, you can draw strength from the memory of someone's stepping in or your finding unexpected strength. Rather than allow a painful past experience to keep you in a state of contraction, you can remember its positive aspects and use them to give you courage.

The mind has the marvelous capacity to experience emotions connected to a prior memory over and over again, each time you recall that memory. When you close your eyes and imagine yourself standing at the shore of a lake, happily tossing in stones with your grandfather at your side, you recreate the feelings of contentment and love. You can use such a wholesome memory as an antidote to emotional pain whenever you feel unloved or insecure.

When a client has an unwholesome self-judgment, I help her experience its wholesome antidote. For example, an interior designer I work with felt that she wasn't unique or special. I knew from our sessions that this belief was holding her back from expanding her business in a creative way, which she needed to do in order to meet the goals she'd set for herself. I asked her to recall a time when she felt unique or special.

Sometimes my clients insist that they never, not for a moment, felt a particular wholesome quality, but I always press this point, because I know that with some effort,

they can find one, however small. I tell the client that it's as if his computer has given him the error message "file not found" because he's searched for it in the wrong area of his hard drive. Through mindfulness meditation, we can recover such moments that the conscious mind has forgotten and "restore the file." Once you find and restore that file, you can reprogram your belief system, consciously choosing to lay a new neural network. However, if you decide to retain that file, you reinforce the old unwholesome belief, ensuring that it will affect your self-image in the future and limiting your opportunities for creative transformation that would lead to deeper fulfillment.

You can return repeatedly to this wholesome memory, all the while using it as a positive antidote. When you do, you'll reinforce a new, consciously chosen, wholesome self-judgment. My client was able to access a memory of putting her senior art project on display for the class, and the tremendous admiration and respect her classmates showered on her. Each time she recalled this memory, it re-created in her feelings of being talented, creative, and special.

Creating a New Memory

Another technique for transforming an unwholesome self-judgment into a wholesome one is to consciously rewrite a traumatic memory. Doing so lessens the intensity of the unwholesome feelings attached to it and lays new neural networks for remembering a positive, enhancing experience (albeit one created in the imagination). By creating this healing memory, you ensure that whenever the original memory arises in your awareness, it won't cause you as much pain as it used to.

A Memory Made Wholesome

After meditating for several minutes, turn your mind's eye to the scene of an upsetting memory, recalling exactly where you were, how you felt, and any sensory experiences you had at the time (remembering the

Cultivate mindfulness, and the witnessing self will arise unexpectedly as you go about your activities.

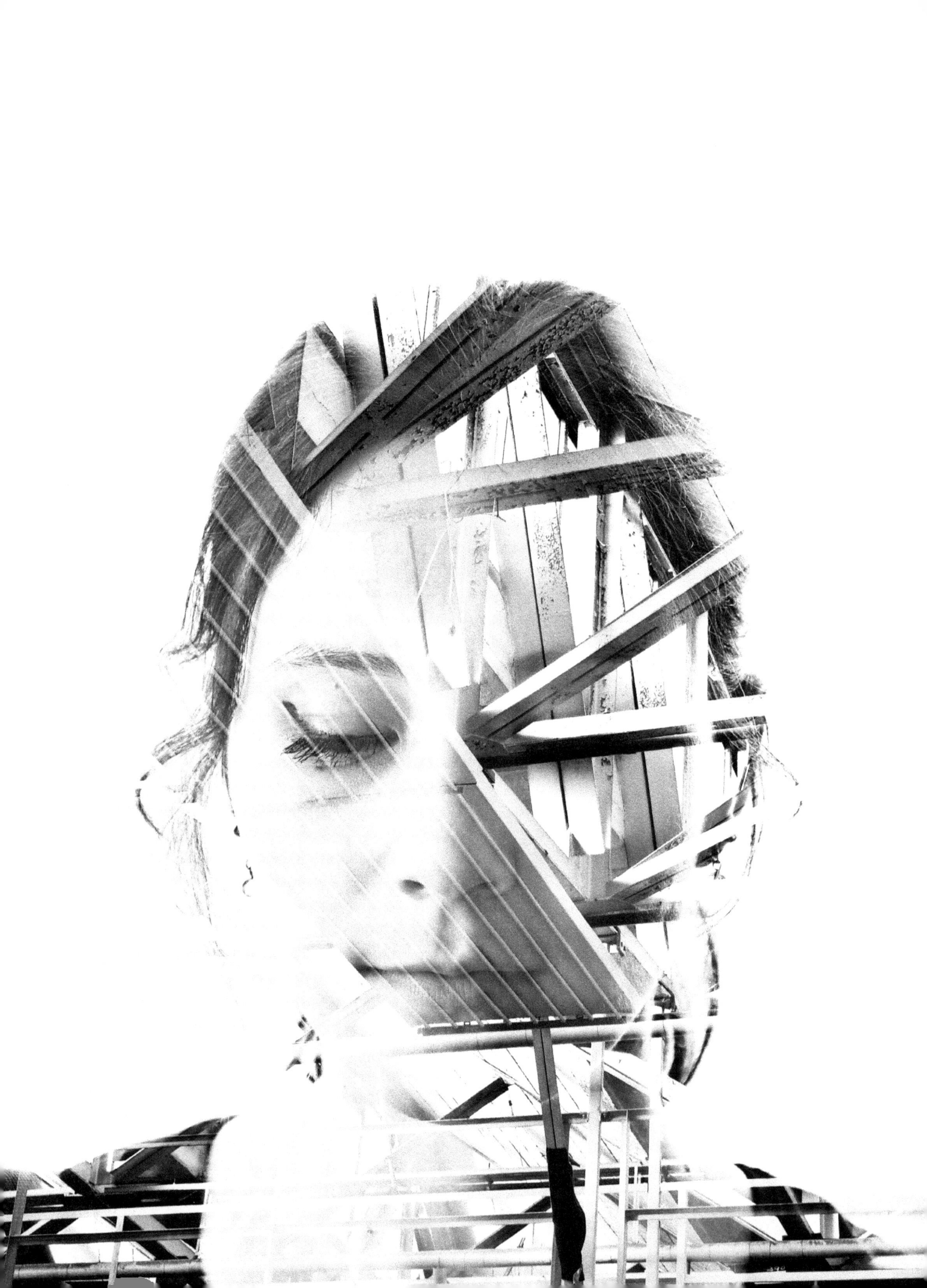

sensory aspects will help you remove any unwholesome feelings that come up when you have similar experiences in the future, for instance, if you usually become agitated when it rains, because you associate it with that unpleasant memory). Put yourself completely in the scene.

As the scene starts to unfold, imagine yourself being drawn upward and backward by an invisible source that deposits you in a balcony seat from which you gaze down at the drama before you. Be aware that you're writing the script of this play, and begin to rewrite it. Imagine that in the moment of your embarrassment, the people around you express support, smiling and encouraging you to continue.

Experience the discomfort of this moment mingling with your rising courage, and allow yourself to breathe deeply. Move the feelings through your body as you rewrite the scene to unfold in a way that alleviates your discomfort and makes you feel reassured of being loved and accepted by the people around you.

Letting Go of the False Self and "Becoming Nobody"

The false self, also called the "ego" or the "egoic mind," is the self we identify with when we're focused on our own needs or importance. The false self is not "bad," but identifying solely with this self, rather than the core self, leads to unwholesome thoughts, feelings, and behaviors. The more we engage in egoic mind, the harder it is to handle a crisis. The ego must move out of the way if we're to immerse ourselves in the three-step process of creative transformation. In the state of open mind, the ego's voice is but a whisper, drowned out by the call of our soul.

The false self is overly influenced by external voices that we internalize, voices that say "You aren't good enough unless you..." or "You'll suffer unless you..." Fear dominates the thinking of the false self and causes us to become self-absorbed, defensive, or overly identified with our roles and situations. When change comes, the false self is alarmed and urges us to resist in an attempt to avoid suffering.

To prevent the false self from taking charge, spiritual teacher Ram Dass suggests the dramatic step of an advanced practice he calls "going into nobody training" (Dass 2007). "Becoming nobody" means letting go of your preconceived notions about your roles and practicing open mind, allowing yourself to discover what's beyond those roles that the false self fiercely clings to, because even the most positive role can limit us and hold us back.

Raised in a prominent Boston family, Richard Alpert knew very early in his childhood that his family expected him to follow in his father's and grandfather's footprints. He went on to become a psychologist and professor at Berkeley and Harvard in the 1960s, but was fired after his experiments with LSD at Harvard. It was a devastating blow, because he was completely identified with being a well-respected psychologist, author, and professor. However, because of LSD, he had experienced open-mind consciousness, so he was ultimately able to break away from this overidentification with the roles he'd played as a psychologist and professor, and let go of his parents' expectations, which had caused him to walk this particular path. Only then was he able to forge a new life as a spiritual teacher, and develop a new identity as Ram Dass. He came to realize that despite all the trappings of success, including having his own private plane and the admiration of his students, his former life had made him profoundly unhappy, an uncomfortable truth he'd avoided facing for years. The crisis of loss made him realize that though the mandala he'd created may have seemed wholesome and good, it didn't represent the calling of his soul. "Becoming nobody," silencing his false self, allowed him to access his core self and form a new, far more fulfilling mandala for himself.

Inside all of us lie possibilities that might

Bring mindful awareness to each and every negative, self-judgmental thought that arises, and watch for a theme to reveal itself.

Becoming nobody means letting go of your preconceived notions about your roles and practicing open mind.

sound preposterous to us in the present moment. To access them, we must undergo the art of creative transformation.

Excerpt from Dr. Ronald Alexander's book, Wise Mind, Open Mind: Finding Purpose and Meaning in Times of Crisis, Loss, and Change. Reprinted with permission: New Harbinger Publications, Inc. Copyright © 2009 Ronald A. Alexander, Ph.D.

Ronald Alexander, Ph.D., is a mind-body psychotherapist, international leadership consultant, and the Executive Director of the OpenMind Training Institute in Santa Monica, a leading-edge organization that offers personal and professional training programs in mind-body therapies, transformational leadership, and mindfulness. He is the author of the widely acclaimed book Wise Mind, Open Mind that provides practical and innovative applications to help us through challenging times. Visit his website: ronaldalexander.com

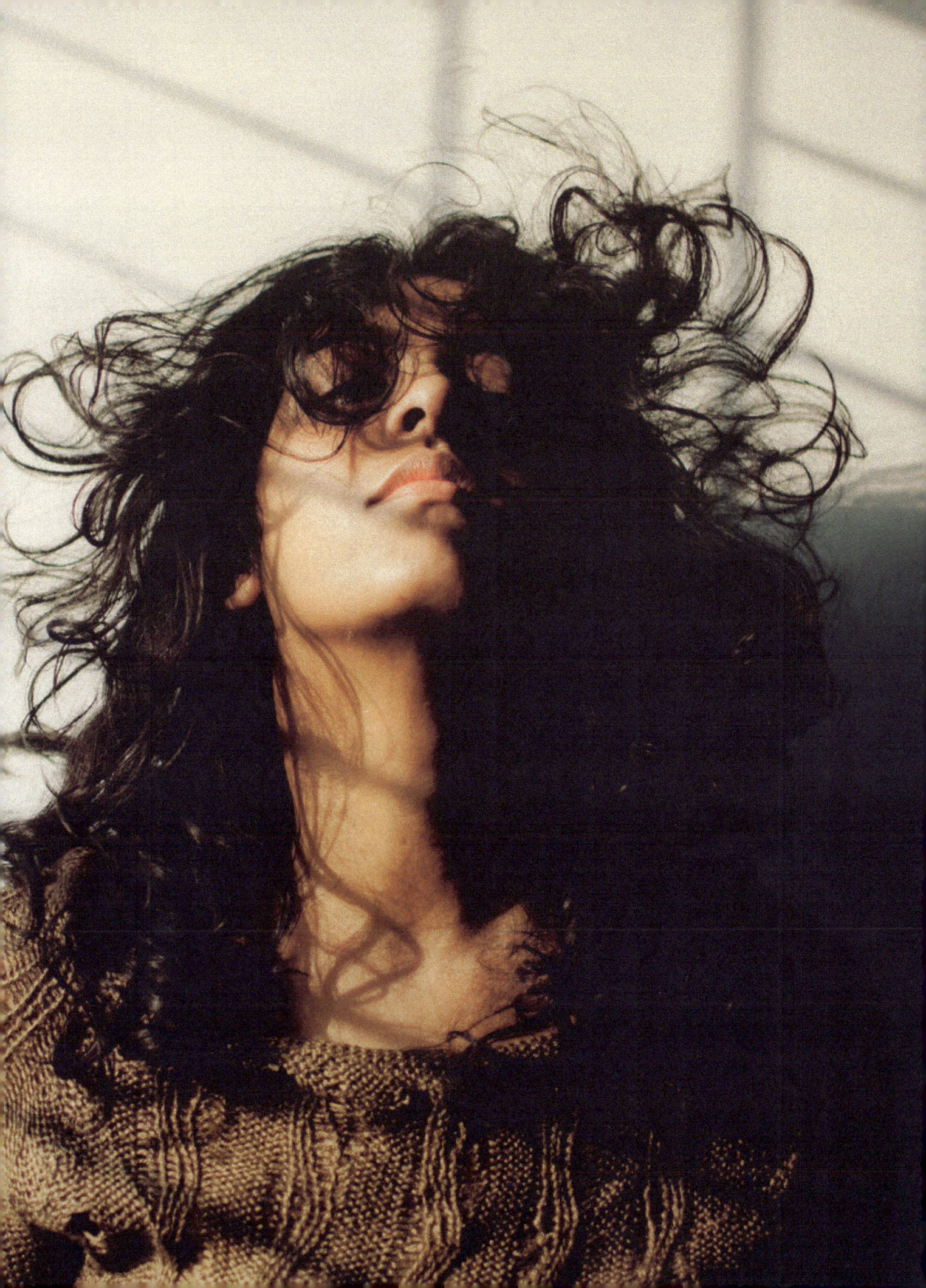

everything in the
universe is within you.
ask all from yourself.

rumi

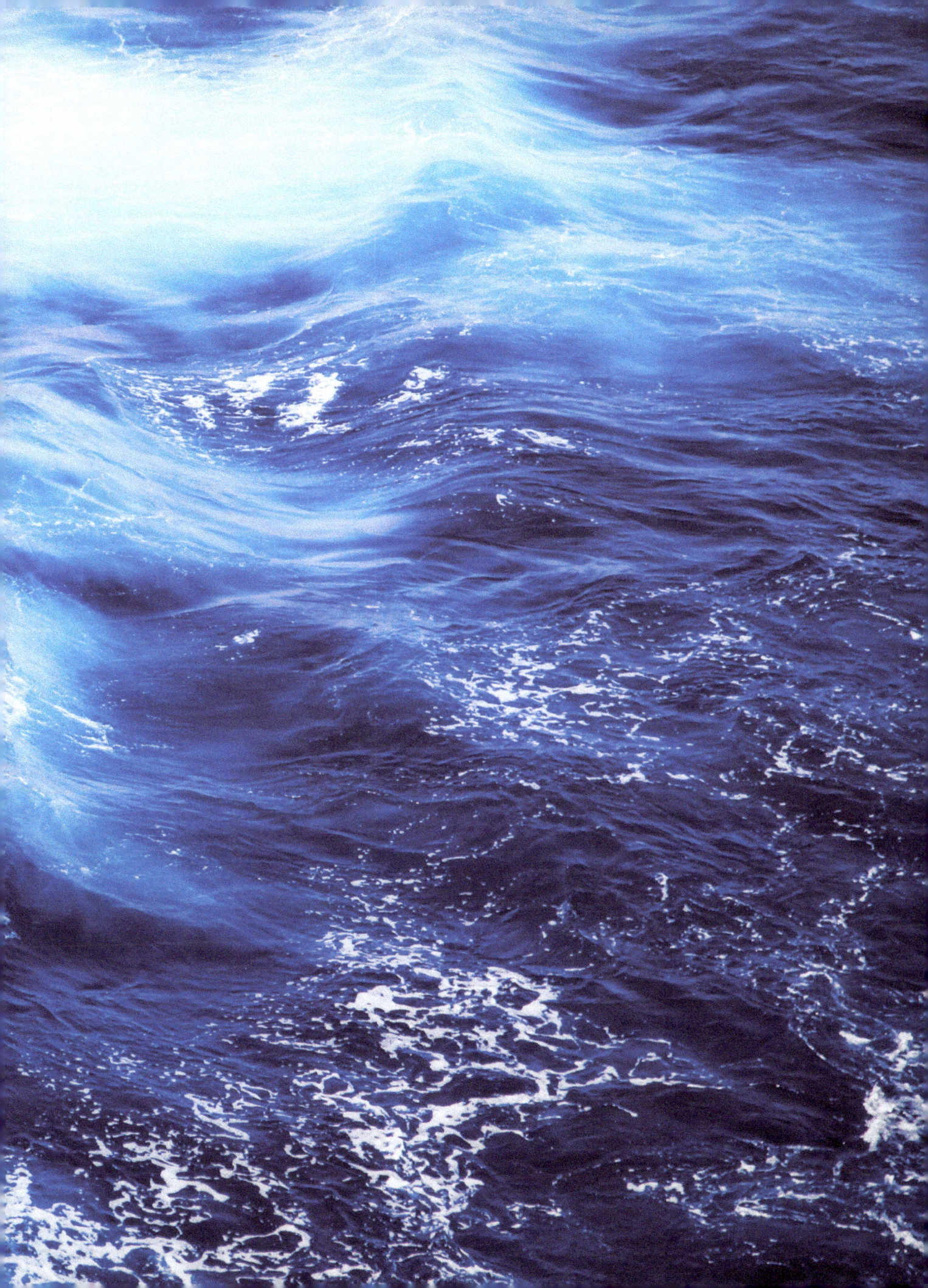

THE PROVIDENCE PROJECT

BEN DECKER IS ON A MISSION TO HEAL THE WORLD WITH MEDITATION

BY JUSTIN FAERMAN + MEGHAN MCDONALD

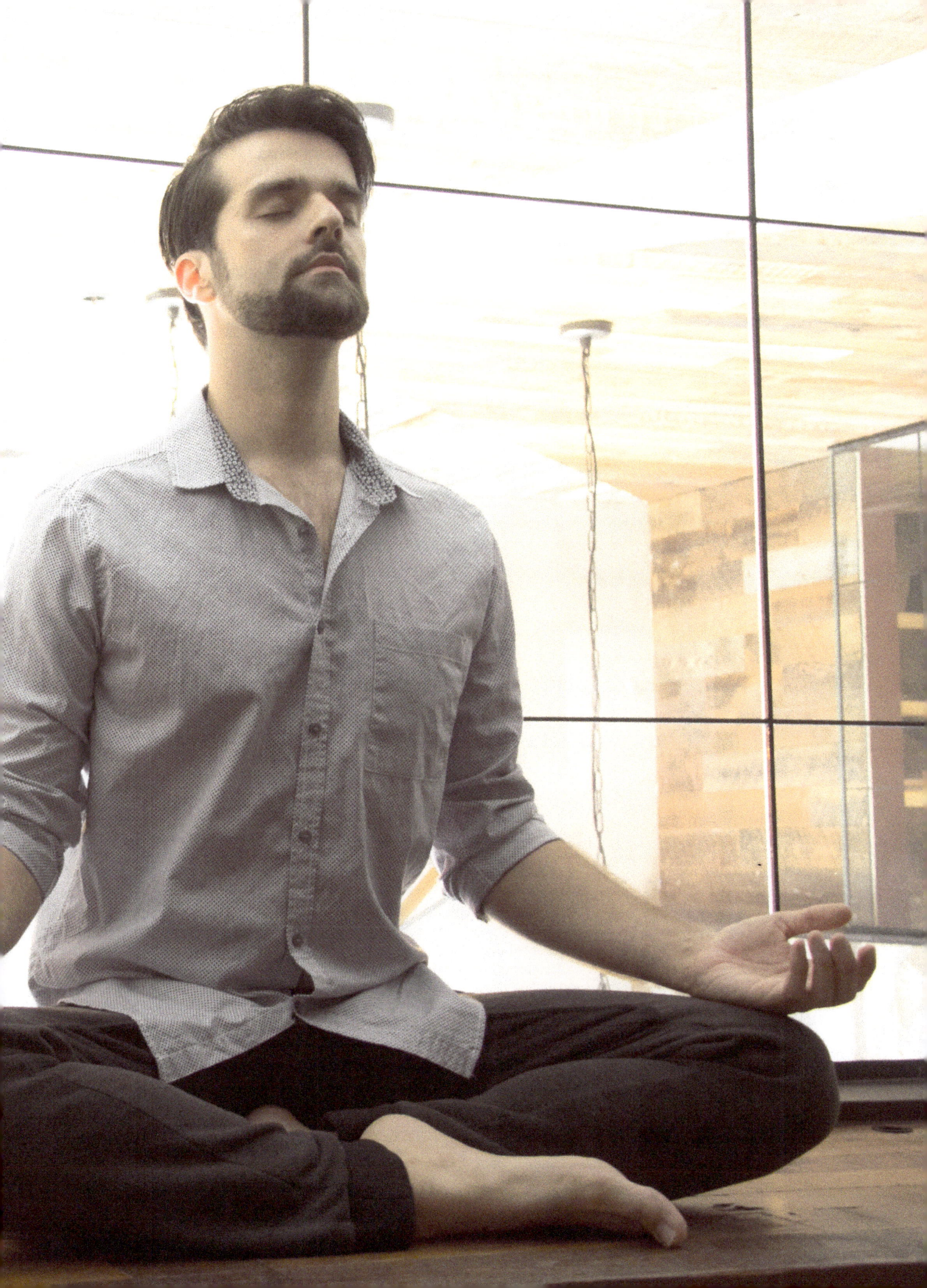

> I was able
> to bear witness
> to the immense
> transformation of
> others through
> the power of
> meditation.

A wise mentor of mine used to say that to understand where life is leading you, connect the dots between where you have been. Following this logic, it becomes quite clear why Ben Decker would undertake the incredibly challenging, but infinitely rewarding path that he has of dedicating his life to transforming our society's most bureaucratic and underserved institutions through meditation and mindfulness. Having experienced its massively transformational power firsthand and witnessing its impact on the lives of others, it became clear that life was indeed leading him somewhere profound.

"There have been many moments in my life where, in meditation, I experienced a direct transition—from addiction to freedom from addiction; from dysfunctional relationships to seeing the way out of dysfunctional relationships; from bearing witness to my own suffering, my own childhood traumas and being able to process through and ultimately overcome them," Ben shared with us during an interview about his burgeoning nonprofit, The Providence Project, which offers meditation and mindfulness training to various institutions and communities, including schools, rehabilitation centers, detention centers, hospitals, and law enforcement officers.

His fascination with the life-altering power of meditation came not just from personal experiences with the practice but from witnessing firsthand its effects on others. "There is one unforgettable incident that I experienced where I was able to bear witness to the immense transformation of others through the power of meditation." He shifted nervously in his seat as he opened up to us: "I've never shared this story publicly until now... When I was on a trip to the Philippines with an anti-human trafficking organization I'd become very involved with, Unlikely Heroes, we were spending a few days working with a group of girls that had been rescued from sex trafficking. Each girl had their own individual story; but, they were all under 18, most under the age of 15, and had been raped

countless times."

The mood in the room grew tense as the story unfolded. Ben recalled that one of the girls had been strangled and left for dead, but was fortunately found and resuscitated. "Encountering these girls, and seeing their social dynamic with each other, it was unmistakably obvious: they were very guarded, they had walls up against each other; they didn't even want to look me in the eye. They had walls up against all of the people that were there to help them, especially the men that were there, myself included."

Ben paused to take a sip of water and collect himself, clearly still moved by his experience many years later. "They had been through very serious, very extreme trauma," he murmured before continuing. After being moved to a safe place, the girls were fed, given gifts, and reassured, but there wasn't much of a change in their demeanor.

"After a series of different activities, we actually sat down and had them close their eyes. We said a prayer with them. We had them just sit there in silence, taking a few deep breaths. In those moments, we let them know that they were in a safe place; that we were there specifically for them and to help them... that they mattered; that their lives mattered; that things that had already happened to them were irrelevant to what was going to happen to them in the future, and that they are powerful; that they could overcome anything. The energy in the room became very still as we sat there in silence. We saw all of the girls—the demeanor of each of these very hard, very tough girls—became very soft and they all suddenly became very vulnerable."

Ben described the scene after the meditation as one of great transformation—the girls were crying and hugging each other—later that day they were playing and singing as if all of that trauma had suddenly evaporated. "It was like a miracle had been performed," he choked. "Even just for that day, they were allowed to just be teenagers again, they were allowed to just be young girls rather than

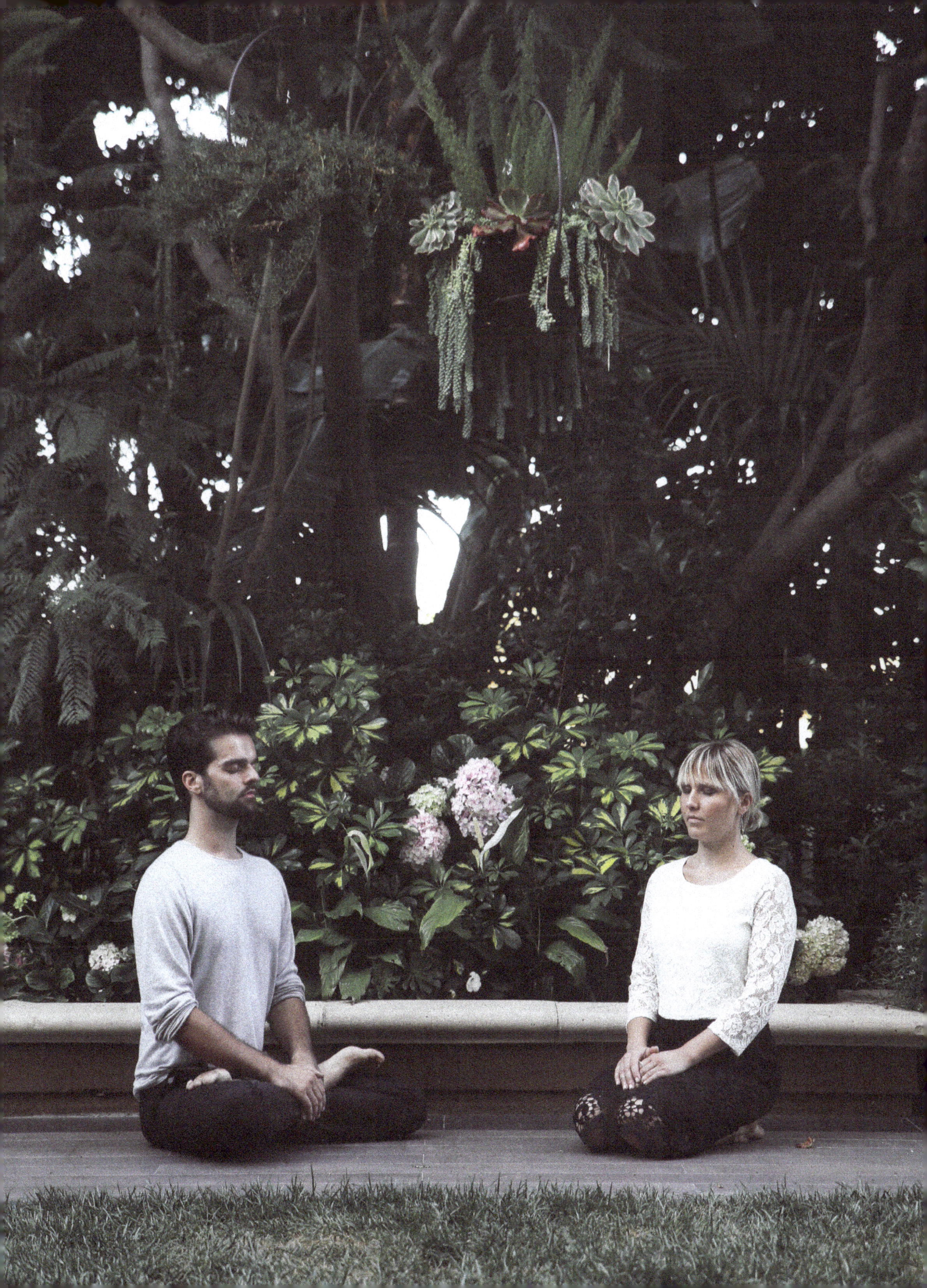

It was so
much bigger
than we ever
could have
imagined that
moment
to be.

having to live through the horror of what had happened to them."

Although reluctant to admit it, it's clear this experience left an indelible mark on his soul.

"It was emotional for me also. It was one of the most magical moments I have ever experienced. I was crying; I had tears in my eyes. All the other adults that were with me, we were all really speechless. It was something very divine; it was so much bigger than we ever could have imagined that moment to be. It was as though something truly divine, truly powerful, had passed through that room. My immediate thoughts were relating that moment to my own life, how I could overcome anything in my own life."

Experiences like these shape our lives in unexpected ways, instantly transforming the way we see ourselves and the world around us. Ben remembers seeing a female police officer a few days later while still in the Philippines, whose demeanor was also characteristic of the same tough exterior and a similar underlying hurt and trauma. "I just started to see it. And, I thought, wow; what if we could provide that moment to police officers? And let them know: Hey, you've got this! You're awesome! We so appreciate what you're doing. And you, as an individual, matter no matter what, if you decided to not be a police officer or if you decide to continue being a police officer."

Swept up in the zeitgeist of his experiences, Ben began to see the pressing need for similar interventions throughout society's most troubled institutions.

"I thought: what if we could provide that healing, transformational moment to people who are in prison, who believe that they're bad and believe that they should be judged for the things that they've done? What if we could start to bring those transformational moments into those places? Would they cry? Would they hug each other after? Would they start laughing with each other after the way these girls did?"

"In the months after that, all these other ideas started to come through," remem-

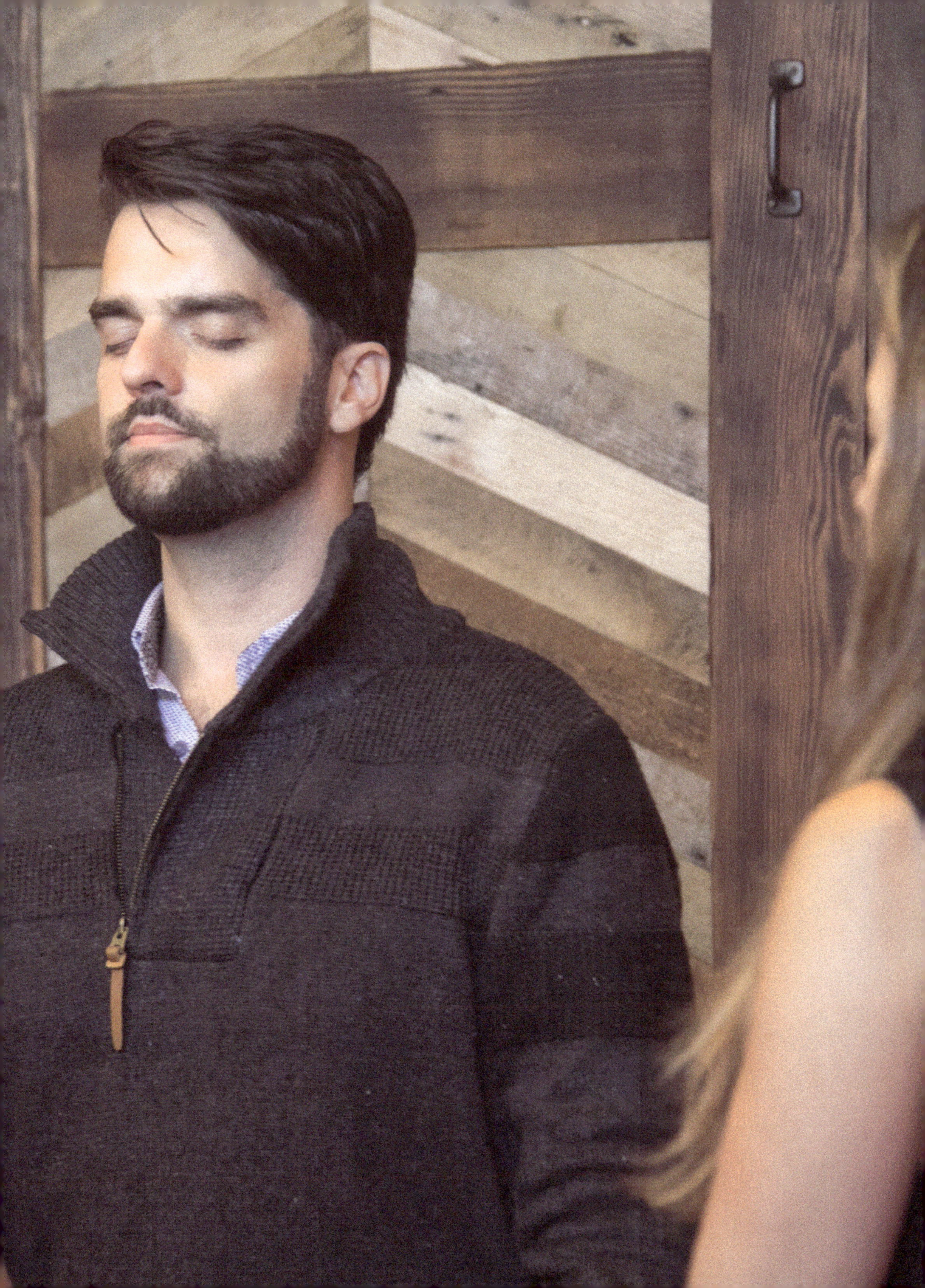

> What would happen if world leaders and politicians had this same experience? Would wars end?

bers Ben. "I started to meet people: cancer patients, AIDS patients, mental health patients—and even just children living their normal lives, with normal upbringings. What if we could provide that moment to children who just feel insecure on their first day of school? They don't even need to have experienced extreme trauma; everyone experiences anxiety and suffering in their own way. What if we were able to just provide that in areas where it could be needed? The transformational potential in that was really inspiring."

Upon his return to the U.S., the inspiration continued to avalanche in. What would happen if everyone could experience something like this? How would society change? What would happen if world leaders and politicians had this same experience? Would wars end? Would major issues find peaceful resolution? Would it trickle down to the masses? "Giving myself that time to dream about that—it was a few months of dreaming—a few months of just, what can I do? I don't know where to begin with this; it was just such a big, lofty dream. And I realized you just kind of start where you are."

What you don't know about Ben is that he knows how to hustle—how to make things happen. The intoxicating dream of becoming an actor lured him out west as a teenager, leaving behind everything that couldn't fit in his car—family, friends and the only life he knew up to that point. Like so many before him, he soon found himself stranded in Los Angeles without a cent to his name. But there was no turning back. It was all or nothing, a proverbial right of passage to discover who he truly was.

When the acting failed to pan out, he quickly discovered he was good at public relations. Really good. Within a few years, he was running a well-staffed PR agency that he had built from scratch, working with some of the world's most well-known brands and a number of burgeoning nonprofits, including Unlikely Heroes, to raise awareness about humanitarian causes closer to his heart. But despite the fame, glamour and success, the unrelenting pressure to perform and the toll it was taking on his life was slowly eating away at his conscience.

"It was a lot of stress—it was a really high stress environment," Ben reflected on his life running the agency. "Everyone around me was constantly having anxiety attacks, and there was a really serious issue with depression. It was constant chaos. My health was deteriorating, my anxiety was off the charts."

"Before I knew it, I had been in LA. for six years and my entire life had been co-opted by the PR industry. I was gaining a lot of weight and aging really rapidly. I had all kinds of health issues coming up left and right. Doctors were shoving medication in my face... I eventually realized that my life wasn't working, and so I began the process of unraveling everything I had spent the last half decade building."

And as is so often the case in these moments of defeat, we find great clarity. Ben's story was no exception. "I was feeling really disconnected and disinterested with life. I was broke and depressed and cynical... even suicidal at times... and then I started meditating. And it changed everything." His face lit up as he recounted the moment, clearly still feeling the emotional ethers of the experience. "I woke up to the reality of my life and realized that it wasn't at all what I wanted, and I just started purging everything negative from my life. Meditation and a handful of close friends saved me from a massively self-destructive trajectory."

And yet, in an ironic twist of fate, it would ultimately be his PR skills, coupled with a newfound self-awareness and meditation practice, that led to the transformational experiences that were his salvation from the unrelenting stress of the entertainment industry.

"After I got back from the Phillipines, I got involved with Marianne Williamson, serving on her campaign for Congress, and through relationships developed by working with her, I began teaching meditation publicly. It was really through that experience of teaching publicly that I started to see how this vision could become something that could pragmatically begin and actually, effectively, be implemented now, right away. So, I decided to create The Providence Project from that place of inspiration to just begin something now." It didn't take long before Ben had developed and implemented free meditation and mindfulness classes across the city. Building on his early successes, he began developing relationships with mental health facilities and other organizations as The Providence Project grew.

His background working closely with charities during his PR days suddenly came into greater focus and found a new form of expression. Instead of raising money for other nonprofits, he's now running his own.

From the very beginning, The Providence Project was different—the ethos was about far more than just raising money for a good cause, it was about transforming society from the roots up—giving the often-marginalized people who need it most a direct experience of the transformation, joy and peace that meditation could bring... just like he experienced with the girls from the Phillipines.

THE BEGINNINGS OF A MOVEMENT

Two years in he's off to a great start. Ben and the project have worked tirelessly to set up regular classes across Los Angeles and are making inroads into many underserved areas of society. Their model is twofold: provide free community classes to anyone looking to learn meditation and mindfulness and serve specific communities by partnering with existing organizations and acting as a social service-enhancement program. By operating in this manner, the classes can be tailored to meet the specific needs of the communities being served.

But despite initial success, it's hardly a walk in the park. Transforming bureaucratic organizations and marginalized communities takes time, patience and fine tuning to meet the specific needs of the people being served.

"We're working with the case managers and everything; hearing what the needs are. Sometimes, for example, if you think it's going to be encouragement these people need, it's not always the case; sometimes you're surprised to find out it's actually anger management; and then we tailor the meditations to really fit what the case managers tell us about the population. And then, once we work with the population, we receive real-time feedback in tailoring that specifically for them," he explained about the intricacies of developing effective programs.

One of his favorite projects to date offers meditation classes to survivors of sex-trafficking in Los Angeles county by working with Saving Innocence—a nonprofit that rescues and advocates for sex-trafficking survivors. As of this writing, Ben and The Providence Project have set up or are in the process of implementing free programs working with police departments, prisons, mental health facilities, rehabilitation centers, school teachers, HIV/AIDS and cancer patients, and virtually everyone in between.

Although the programs have generally been well-received, they face unique challenges with people who don't understand meditation or have preconceived notions about what it is. "There's some people that believe it's a religious practice—there are people who are misinformed about the different types of meditation, and there's also a members-only-club mentality about this type of meditation is better than that type of meditation." On top of this, there's the ingrained belief in our society that doing more is better, and slowing down is a sign of weakness. "Convincing someone like a police officer or politician to sit quietly for a session can take some finesse. There's not only overcoming some of the ignorance and confusion surrounding what the actual work is but also being able to calmly and effectively communicate what the clinically proven benefits are to get someone to the point where they say: OK; I understand meditation; I understand what this is, and I'm open to trying it."

I was broke and depressed and cynical... even suicidal at times... and then I started meditating.

My expectations are really high. There's no limit to what one individual can create and experience.

Which is why The Providence Project has adopted a hybrid, science-backed form of meditation that transcends traditional definitions and stereotypes of the practice: "The method that we use in The Providence Project is based on what has been clinically proven to be effective. So, it has its roots in both Vedic and Buddhist mindfulness meditation, which have a lot of similarities with Kabbalistic meditation and other forms of meditation; but, primarily, it is a mindfulness-based practice."

While The Providence Project doesn't use traditional mantra in the meditations, they still teach about them, along with the various types and styles of meditation. "I really like to teach about the different kinds of meditation, so people can find out what really resonates for them and learn more about that. What we are teaching directly is a totally secular, non-spiritual exercise to connect with your body, take inventory of your body and become aware of the thoughts that are coming through your mind. It's very similar to mindfulness in that way, and it's technically based on mindfulness, but we also use very foundational, fundamental techniques that are not considered to be part of any specific lineage exclusively."

And Ben should know. In addition to running The Providence Project full time, he currently teaches meditation at various locales in Los Angeles, including Wanderlust Hollywood and Unplug Meditation, and works with a number of private clients looking to go deeper in their own practice. His intimacy with the art is a big part of the organization's success, encoding the entire project with deep roots in an experiential, non-dogmatic model. A model that is also designed to be highly scalable—perhaps a reflection of the open-source ethos characteristic of Ben's generation. "The programs are organized in such a way that they are easy to duplicate; the model was created to be reproducible," he chimed when asked about the project's evolution and development.

In order to restructure the fabric of society and have the widest possible impact, The Providence Project will eventually take on a life of its own, meaning that volunteers around the world will be able to form their own spinoff groups based on a shared common methodology and system currently being developed by Ben and his colleagues. "I think that what the world needs and what The Providence Project needs is really committed people," says Ben. "The best way to contribute is to take an inventory of what you do with your life; everyone can help in their own way. You are helping because you have the magazine; you're helping by getting the word out there." In addition to spreading awareness, The Providence Project is particularly focused on finding and training facilitators across the country and world and connecting them with groups in their area that can benefit from meditation. "We can provide the training for how to teach meditation. We can even connect you with groups in your area that need the work and coordinate all of that," he explained. "More than anything, I just want to see the programs grow and thrive with a team of really committed people."

When asked about the future of the Project, Ben is optimistic. "I've already seen so much transformation that my hopes and my vision are very high. In fact, my expectations are really high. There's no limit to what one individual can create and experience. Knowing that and then providing a tool that can actually help an individual recognize that in themselves, we open ourselves up to a world where anything actually is possible."

And in the end, like everything, it all comes full circle.

To learn more about The Providence Project visit their website: theprovidenceproject.org

All photographs shot on location at Wanderlust Hollywood and the Four Seasons Hotel, Beverly Hills.

Justin Faerman & Meghan McDonald *are the founders of Conscious Lifestyle Magazine.*

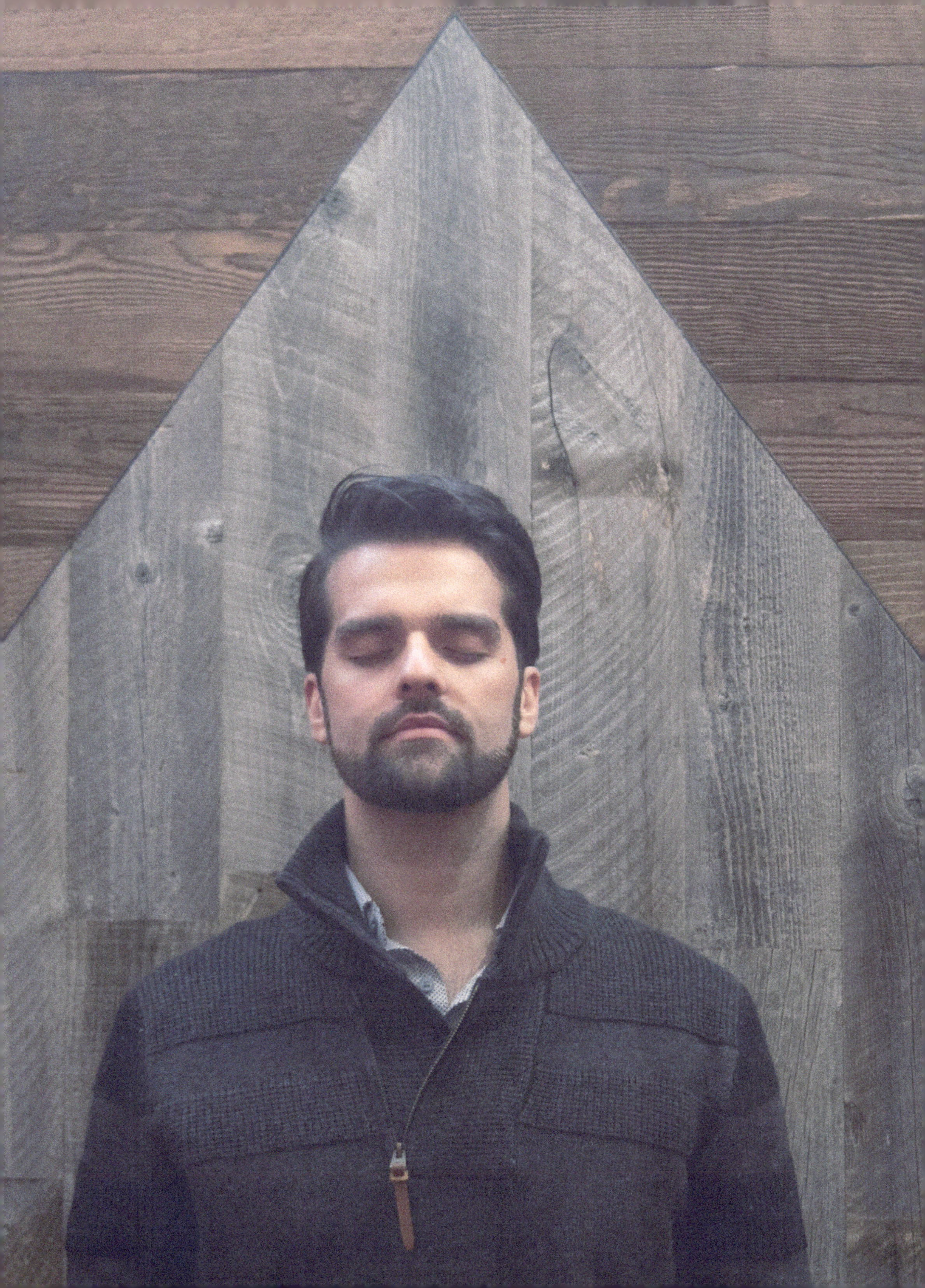

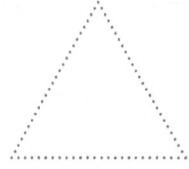

THRIVE

THE 7 CORE QUALITIES OF THE WORLD'S MOST HAPPY & SUCCESSFUL PEOPLE

DONNA STONEHAM, Ph.D.

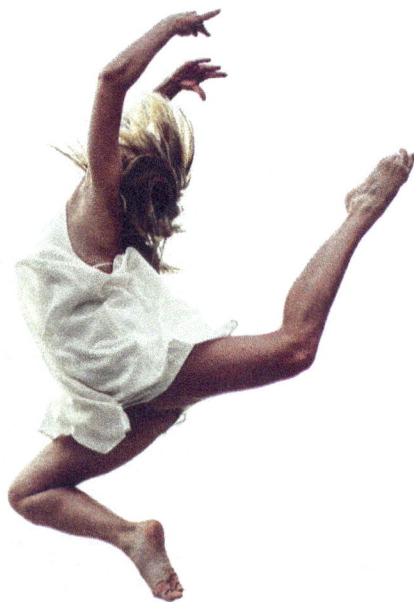

"I don't want to get to the end of my life and find that I have lived just the length of it. I want to have lived the width of it as well."
— **Diane Ackerman**

What does it mean to thrive? How do people who thrive perceive and interact with the world differently from those who settle or live in a state of survival? What does it take to move from one state to the other? These pivotal questions have guided my work and life for twenty-five years.

As a teenager and young adult, I suffered from a debilitating depression that nearly took my life. I lived under a dark cloud of despair that I fought hard to survive throughout my early twenties. As a child, I felt like a stranger in a strange land. I didn't fit in. I was very sensitive and felt things deeply. I often felt misunderstood and had few peers to whom I could relate. At an early age, I began comparing myself to others, was consumed by shame, and believed myself unworthy of being loved. Yet even in the midst of what often felt like unbearable suffering, the part of me that was whole, true, and essential yearned to thrive. There was a "knower" deep inside me who believed thriving was possible, as reflected in this excerpt from a poem I wrote at age fifteen.

I yearn only for a peace which smiles,
To be happy as I walk the miles.
Just simple strength to ease the load
While traveling down life's lonely road.
Mere hope and courage do I ask
To be the doer of my task.
I want to live a life that's free
From pain and its inequity.
To look beneath this wretched me
Open my heart, gaze in to see
A boundless treasure, a priceless wealth
Of love and compassion within myself.
To reach perfect beauty as a rose,
To watch this spirit soar and grow
With lovely wings as I aspire
To reach unknown heights I will acquire.

Thank you, God, for what shall be,
For I shall live and will be free.

At the time I wrote the poem, what I knew in my heart but lacked the life experience to understand was that freedom from shame and self-recrimination was my personal key to thriving. At the heart of this freedom are universal traits that I've discovered that people who thrive possess: self-acceptance, the courage to face our doubts and fears, and the willingness to hold those parts of ourselves we're ashamed of with compassion. As we develop these three capacities, we cultivate a thriver's mindset. At its foundation, this way of perceiving and interacting with the world is built on our ability to cultivate a belief in ourselves, a trust that life will support us, and a faith in something larger to sustain us, however we define that.

The mindset of a thriver also includes an ability to trust in the "flow" of life rather than always needing to try to control it. We have to learn to hold things lightly, rather than grasping tightly to outcomes we feel compelled to achieve. People who thrive develop the capacity to perceive life through a lens of possibilities and opportunities rather than through a filter of obstacles and limitations. They look for why things can happen, rather than why they can't. And thriving necessitates the ability to be present to what's happening in the moment, rather than worrying about the future or ruminating over the past.

THRIVING VERSUS SURVIVING

Many of us carry wounds or traumatic experiences from childhood that influence our sense of worthiness, our belief in ourselves and our capabilities. The statistics on trauma are staggering. Though rates of incidents appear to be decreasing, recent studies claim that 25 to 50 percent of children around the world suffer from physical abuse, and 20 percent of girls and 5 to 10 percent of boys will be sexually abused during childhood. Globally, 35 percent of women have experienced

As a child, I felt like a stranger in a strange land. I didn't fit in. I was very sensitive and felt things deeply.

The mindset of a thriver also includes an ability to trust in the "flow" of life.

physical and/or sexual intimate partner violence or non-partner sexual violence. In 2012, more than 10 percent of children in the U.S. lived with a parent with alcohol problems, while seventeen million adults in the U.S. suffered from alcohol addiction. Mental illness affects one in four American adults each year. Few people are untouched by some kind of challenge or trauma in our lives, but whatever our cross is to bear, if we choose to allow the labels of "victim" or "survivor" to define us and our view of our capabilities, we do so at our own peril.

In my case, perceiving myself as a victim narrowed my perspective and kept me from taking risks. It made me believe I wasn't worthy of creating the life I yearned for, and it caused me to doubt myself. When we label ourselves and allow our past experiences to define the life we live now, we abdicate our power and limit ourselves from becoming all we were meant to become. It's not the challenging experiences we accrue in our lives but rather how we use them as opportunities to transform ourselves that are the hallmark of people who thrive.

BEING PRESENT IN THE MOMENT

Celia, a director at a technology company in the Midwest, is one such woman I worked with who emerged from the fires of past trauma. By shifting the image she'd held of herself and changing what she focused on, she transformed herself from a survivor into a thriver. At the core of her being, Celia yearned to flourish in her job and life, but she didn't know how to get there. When we began our work together, I suggested that she practice being mindful of the differences in her feelings and thoughts in those moments when she experienced herself thriving, as compared with those times when she felt that she was settling or surviving. I asked her to notice what was possible in both states of mind, and how they differed. How did she engage with others? What did she focus on? What results did she create?

After Celia reflected on these questions for two months against the backdrop of her life, I asked what she had learned. She said, "This practice has proven quite revealing. My mind is in a really different space when I'm thriving, both at work and at home. I feel more energized. I don't feel anxious. I feel confident that I can do what needs to get done. I'm not always second-guessing myself."

As Celia continued to name the differences between how she felt when she was thriving versus surviving, three distinctions emerged. First, when she was thriving, she felt present to what was happening in her life at that moment, whether that was having a conversation with her children, working with a colleague, or meeting with one of her clients. She was able to stay focused on what was directly in front of her, rather than thinking about what was ahead or behind. She didn't allow herself to be distracted or derailed by other things or people vying for her attention.

But when she found herself in a survival mindset, Celia allowed her anxiety to divert her attention away from where it was needed in the moment. She found herself worrying about the future or focusing on something that hadn't gone well in the past, which resulted in self doubt. For example, in a recent meeting with her peers, she said, "I found myself holding back from making comments, worried they would judge them as not being valuable to the group." Her fear caused her to become contracted and disconnected from herself and others. She found herself silencing her voice and withholding valuable contributions. When she was functioning in survival mode, she said, "I noticed I give away my power."

TRUST AND ACCEPTANCE

The second distinction Celia made was that when she was thriving, she felt a deeper sense of trust in life and in herself. "I just had faith that things would work out," she said, "and trusted that everything would be okay." When she was able to maintain this mindset of trusting in the "flow" of life, even when things didn't go as planned, she didn't allow herself to get knocked off-center. She just took a deep breath, grounded herself, and moved on.

"I just felt a sense of trust in myself that whatever came my way, I could manage. When I focused on what was going well in my life, I stopped stressing so much about what wasn't working," Celia reported. "When I stopped being so attached to what I thought the outcome ought to be or about what others thought I *should* be doing, and paid more attention to the places where I could make a difference, it was so much easier to accept whatever came my way."

For example, Celia recounted that there were a number of projects she was responsible for that were all due within a short time frame. "In the past," she said, "I used to get myself all worked up about how I would be able to get everything done and spent more energy on worrying than I did on accomplishing things. This time, I decided to take a different approach and trust that I would get everything completed. I looked for ways to be smarter about how I was doing things, and I asked for help from others, whereas before I would have tried to do it all myself. I looked back on my track record over the past few years and realized I always make it happen. So I asked myself, 'Why am I wasting so much of my energy worrying about getting things done?'"

FOCUS ON OPPORTUNITIES AND POSSIBILITIES

What Celia was describing is the third competency that thrivers learn to put into practice. Rather than focusing on the obstacles and limitations in their path, they look instead for ways to do things more effectively. They dismantle the obstacles that keep them from offering their greatest contributions. Instead of looking for all the reasons why things might not happen, thrivers hold a sense of positive expectancy, a faith that good

things will occur, and a belief that they are worthy to receive them. This allows energy to be channeled in productive ways, rather than allowing a belief in limitations to pervade. Recent studies on the neurochemistry of the brain show that when we're thinking negatively about something, our cortisol (stress hormone) level increases, which causes us to be more sensitive and reactive and reduces our ability to think as quickly or creatively.

I remember a powerful quote I heard once: "Worrying is praying for things you don't want." Thrivers maintain an expansive view of themselves and the world. They focus their energy on being open to opportunities and possibilities, rather than worrying about all the things that might go wrong.

The way thrivers experience life depends not on their circumstances, but on the ways they chose to respond to the hand they are dealt. What, for example, enabled Jonah, a common shopkeeper, to become a prophet and save a city? With the odds so stacked against her, what allowed Oprah Winfrey—an impoverished, abused girl from rural Mississippi—to become one of the most inspirational women in the world? What spurred a Viktor Frankl, a Jew dehumanized in a Nazi death camp, to emerge from that experience to write one of the most insightful books of the twentieth century? And what enables people like my client Celia, you, and me to learn to spread our wings and thrive?

The French philosopher Henri-Louis Bergson said, "The eye sees only what the mind is prepared to comprehend." It takes developing the mindset of a thriver in order to become all that we are capable of becoming. What makes this mindset possible is our ability to unlock and use seven key capacities. These include the capacity to trust, to act with humility, to cultivate resilience, to learn to listen to our inner direction, to follow our vision, to assume an attitude of expansiveness, and to take responsibility for the choices we make.

> Thrivers hold a sense of positive expectancy, a faith that good things will occur.

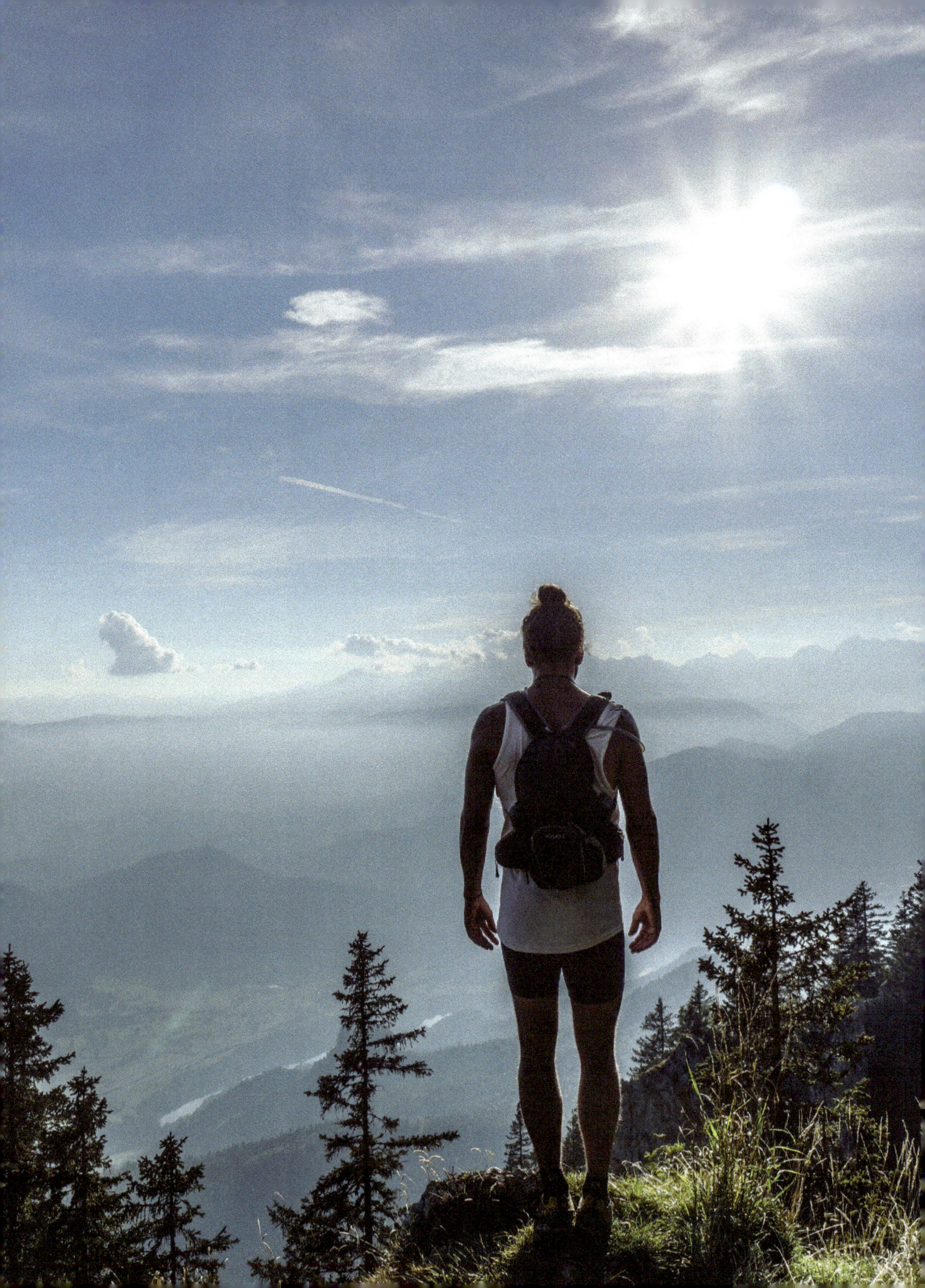

THE SEVEN KEYS TO BECOMING A THRIVER

Trust: Have faith you're never traveling alone.
Humility: Navigate with confident humility.
Resilience: Choose the right bus.
Inner Direction: Follow your compass, it won't fail you.
Vision: Walk into your vision, one step at a time.
Expansiveness: Broaden your horizons.
Responsibility: Be accountable for your choices.

TRUST: THE FIRST KEY

In order to thrive, we must cultivate a trusting spirit. This means developing the faith that life will support us and provide the experiences we need to help us navigate whatever comes our way. It means trusting ourselves and our inner "knower" to take the right next step in our lives, rather than allowing our actions to be prescribed by others' expectations or by our own insecurities. It means trusting ourselves to have the courage to step into the unknown, even without a guarantee of what lies around the next bend. And finally, it's about having faith in the basic goodness of others, despite past betrayals or negative experiences that may cause us to doubt this is true.

HUMILITY: THE SECOND KEY

Second, we have to develop true humility: the kind of humility in which we have confidence in our abilities without becoming self-inflated. We cultivate humility as we develop patience and build our capacity to be present with whatever is happening around us. Being present enables us to listen deeply to others, to respond to their needs, and to acknowledge and act on the deepest yearnings within ourselves. True humility is grounded in compassion and kindness for ourselves and for others, which enables us to be both vulnerable and authentic. Having compassion for ourselves means we learn how to step beyond self-imposed limitations by heeding the voice of our inner champion. In order to thrive, we also have to learn to be kind to those parts of ourselves we feel ashamed of, just as a loving parent would care for a frightened child. We learn to embrace, rather than resist, the parts of ourselves that were injured, while not allowing those wounds to dictate the choices we make or to take away our power. In order to express true humility, we have to learn how to love and accept ourselves as the imperfect beings we are.

RESILIENCE: THE THIRD KEY

Developing resilience also helps us thrive, even in times of great challenge. We build this capacity by taking care of ourselves and regularly refilling our well so we are able to bounce back quickly from life's challenges and defeats. To thrive, we have to develop self-mastery in ways that allow us to listen and respond to the inner signals that tell us when it's time to create, when it's time to rest, when it's time to play, and when it's time to nurture our spirits. We can't contribute our best if we're depleted, just as we can't help a child on an airplane without first putting on our own oxygen mask. Setting appropriate boundaries and taking care of our bodies, our spirits, and our emotions with regular self-care practices help us stay focused, grounded, and healthy. These practices are critical in nurturing the resilience it takes to sustain the capacity to live on the thriver's edge.

INNER DIRECTION: THE FOURTH KEY

Our ability to thrive is also predicated on our ability to be inner-directed. It requires that we find the courage to break the cultural trance that says we have to acquire more, be smarter, work harder, be more conniving and more resourceful than the person next door. In order to be true to ourselves and appreciate that we are enough just as we are, we have to learn to stop judging and comparing ourselves

The way thrivers experience life depends not on their circumstances, but on the ways they chose to respond to the hand they are dealt.

> True humility is grounded in compassion and kindness for ourselves and for others.

to others. We can value others' achievements, but we need to learn not to beat ourselves up with a set of should-haves, could-haves, or would-haves.

Comparing ourselves to others can cause us to feel diminished, unworthy, or insecure—or, conversely, to feel that we are better than others. These judgments separate us from being our best and keep us distanced from one another. We all have a path to greatness, yet each of those paths is unique. Learning to listen to the voice of our inner "knower," and to follow the call of our heart, are things that thrivers do well.

VISION: THE FIFTH KEY

Being a thriver requires vision. Thriving doesn't depend on a roll of the dice. It's a creative act. Painting a rich and vibrant life on a blank canvas requires intention, grace, surrender, and will, all in proper balance. But first we have to devote the space and time it takes to envision the life we're being called to express. There is a clear and compelling purpose for every life, yet many of us rarely take the time to be still, to listen, and to reflect on what that purpose is. Those of us fortunate enough even to have the privilege to ask the question Why am I here? must be patient for the answer and have faith that if we listen long enough, our mission will be revealed. Learning to be present to ourselves, to those we care about, and to the world around us helps make this revelation possible.

EXPANSIVENESS: THE SIXTH KEY

Cultivating the mindset of the thriver requires a deep commitment to our continued expansion and evolution, and it takes a dedication to lifelong learning. It is not a straight-line path, but a spiral that involves a circuitous journey round and back and round again. And with each time around the spiral, our wisdom is deepened by our openness to try new things, to take more risks, and to question our assumptions. To thrive means saying "yes" to life and new experiences. It requires

we develop the capacity to live in the present moment while being open to what life delivers and willing to explore its many facets. In order to thrive, we have to take risks to step into the unknown. Thriving requires that we ask a very different set of questions and begin to focus on what we are being asked to give to the world rather than get what we can from it.

RESPONSIBILITY:
THE SEVENTH KEY

Finally: In order to thrive, we have to take action. We must take responsibility for our conditions, whatever they are, and make a commitment to change them if we desire to have a different life. We have to be willing, as the Serenity Prayer says, to "change the things we can" and to not depend on those around us to make our situation better. Taking responsibility for our lives means accepting personal accountability for the choices we make and the life we've created, rather than blaming others for what we don't have or haven't yet accomplished. We may possess the most compelling vision in the world, but if we aren't willing to brave the challenges we encounter while trying to bring that vision into reality, we will never fulfill our potential. We have the ability to make our mark in the world, or we wouldn't have been given the aspiration. It's our response to our abilities that separates thrivers from those who limit themselves.

Thriving is our birthright as human beings. Many of us have just forgotten how to do it because we've gotten lost on the road of comparison. We've grown so accustomed to focusing on what the traveler walking next to us has that we want, that we've lost who we are in the process. Becoming a thriver takes patience and practice. It requires courage, grace, and developing a level of comfort with ambiguity and not knowing. But its rewards far outweigh its effort and struggle. Becoming a thriver is the greatest gift we can give ourselves, extend to those we love, and bequeath to a world in need of transformation.

REFLECTION QUESTIONS AND PRACTICES FOR DEVELOPING THE MINDSET OF A THRIVER

1. In what situations and with whom do you feel most trusting? What makes that possible? In what places in your life would it benefit you to be more trusting and less controlling? How so? What would enable you to trust more readily in the flow of life? If you were able to be more trusting, how would it change your life?

2. How much of your time are you able to be present in the moment rather than think about the future or the past? How would your life be different if you could focus more of your energy on being present in the moment?

3. In all honesty, do you hold a glass-half-empty or a glass-half-full perspective on the world? How open are you to seeing opportunities and possibilities? What is one belief you hold about yourself that is limiting you from expressing more of your potential? What belief could you replace that limiting belief with that would help you create a more expansive, vibrant life? How would it help you thrive?

AN INVITATION TO PRACTICE: BUILDING YOUR CAPACITY TO THRIVE

Look at the seven keys to thriving (trust, humility, resilience, inner direction, vision, expansiveness, and responsibility). Which one is the easiest for you to experience, and which is most difficult? Examine the quality you best exemplify in your work and life. What makes that possible? What have you learned about yourself as you've demonstrated that quality? Identify lessons learned, and look for ways to apply your learning to the qualities you are seeking to develop.

Over the next month, pick the quality from that list that you find most challenging.

Every day, practice getting a little better at it. For instance, if you need to work on trusting more deeply and letting go of the need to control, give a job that you normally would do yourself to your child, your spouse, or someone at work, and let the other person do it. Resist the urge to tell them what to do or how to do it. Notice what happens to you and to the relationship when you're able let go. Each day, stretch yourself to deepen the quality you are seeking to develop. Notice how doing so deepens your ability to be present, to see possibilities, and to cultivate a deeper sense of trust.

AN INVITATION TO PRACTICE: BUILDING COURAGE TO CHANGE AND GROW

For the next few weeks, practice doing one thing each day that pushes you a little further outside your comfort zone. Each day, make a conscious choice to up the ante on the challenge. Start small and build. For some, this may mean setting a boundary with someone with whom you're afraid to set limits. For others, it may mean picking up the phone and calling someone whose help you need in order to take the next step in your life that your intuition is telling you to take. Notice what happens when you face your fears and walk through them. Write in your journal what you learn about yourself and your capacity to express courage as you continue to engage in this practice. Aim high. Who knows where it might take you?

This article is excerpted with permission from The Thriver's Edge: Seven Keys to Transform the Way You Live, Love, and Lead by Donna Stoneham.

Donna Stoneham, Ph.D., *is an executive coach, transformational leadership consultant, and educator, helping hundreds of Fortune 1000 and non-profit leaders, teams & organizations unleash their power to thrive. Visit her website: donnastoneham.com*

> Thriving is our birthright as human beings. Many of us have just forgotten how to do it.

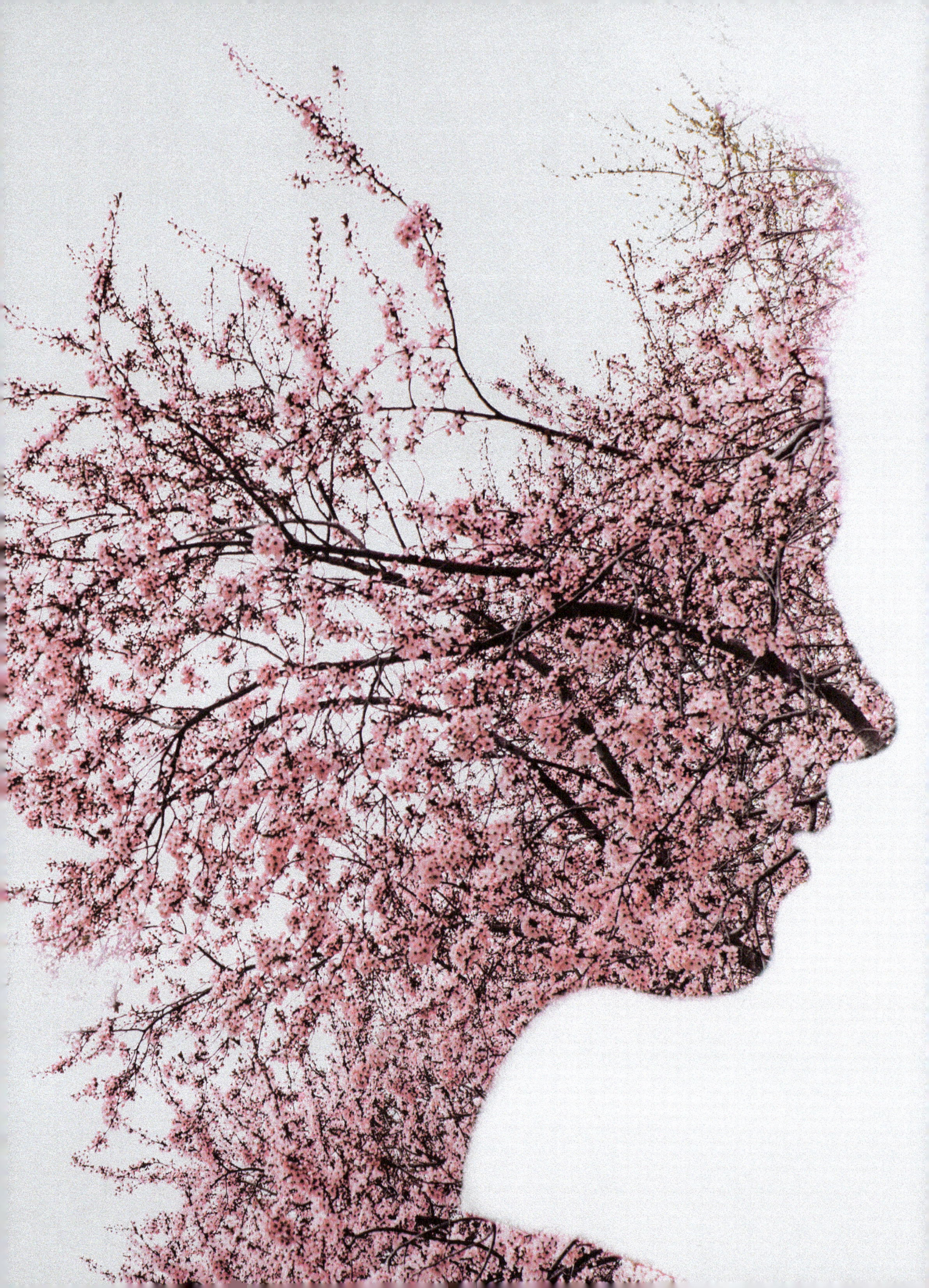

QUANTUM EVOLUTION

HOW TO MAKE BIG, POSITIVE SHIFTS IN YOUR HAPPINESS AND PROSPERITY

by cynthia sue larson

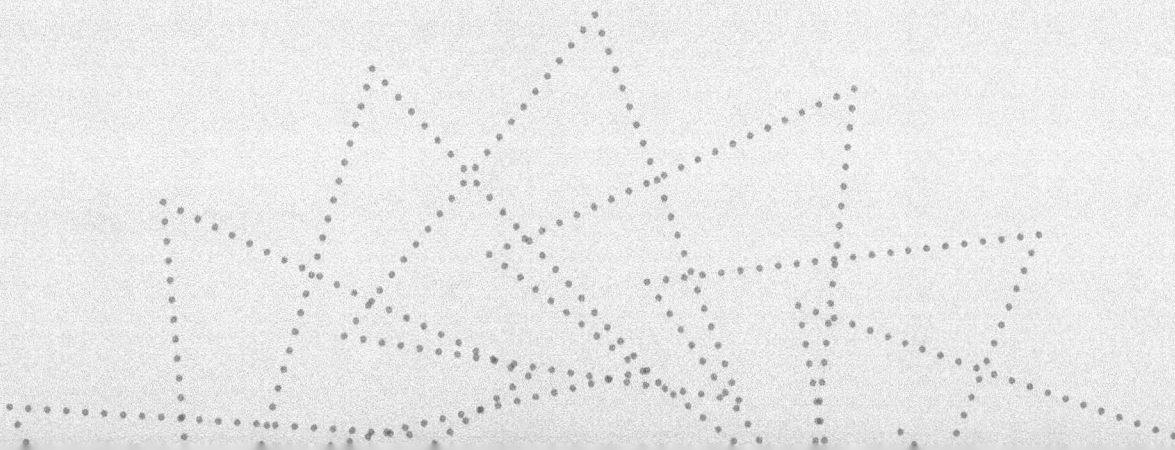

Some quantum jumps can literally be leaps to a better future.

WHAT ARE QUANTUM JUMPS?

The popular expression "quantum jump" is used in common English speech to describe a leap that is big—but to physicists, quantum jumps are tiny, discrete (indivisible), and abrupt. The idea of quantum particles is that they can exist in material form at one energy level or another, but not in between. When quantum particles are observed to make a quantum jump from one state to another, scientists watch them appear to blink on and off.

Quantum jumping is the process by which a person envisions some desired result or state of being that is different from the existing situation—and by clearly observing that possibility and supplying sufficient energy, makes a leap into that alternate reality. The idea behind quantum jumping is that we are living in a multiverse of parallel universes. Usually, these alternate realities have no connection to one another. A quantum jump can be made through a kind of handshake through time and space—this connection forms a bridge that allows someone experiencing a quantum jump to physically end up in another reality. The connection is so total that a person can literally walk into another place and time. While to the universe, both of "you" still exists, your awareness of who you are coalesces in one reality, often leaving the other out of reach, out of sight, and out of mind.

Does any of this seem outlandish or too far-out to be real? While quantum jumping may at first sound like an idea from science fiction, this term actually covers a wide range of experiences from the rather mundane to the truly extraordinary.

As you learn more about various examples of quantum jumps, you'll likely recognize common experiences from your daily life when you've made quantum jumps—often without realizing it at the time.

Imagine the example of a child who receives a mother's kiss after falling down and skinning a knee who suddenly feels much better...or any of a number of clinical trial participants with headaches who, upon taking a placebo (such as a sugar pill), is amazed to find a terrible headache suddenly gone. Visualize another example of a man preparing for an interview by dressing for success... in attire worn by those making the hiring decisions.

In these examples, we find no material-based reason for why the child and clinical study participant are feeling much better and the interviewee feeling so much more confident and self-assured; but chances are very good that we've felt such inexplicably dramatic improvements many times in our lives over the years.

Some quantum jumps can literally be leaps to a better future, as seen in the real-life example of Ashley Clouse's ten-foot leap to safety in the face of an oncoming tornado. We are capable of taking hundreds of quantum leaps in any given day, making decisions that seem inconsequential or small at the time, yet have the collective power to entirely transform our lives. A daily decision to spend a few minutes writing, exercising, or practicing music makes a tremendous difference in a person's life over a period of weeks, months, and years.

In most cases, people experience walking into parallel worlds that are nearly—but not quite entirely—identical to the one they came from. In such cases, it is possible to find something has seemingly shifted in some startling way. A door or building may appear where one had not been before, or you might notice your keys are not where you left them...and after searching for a while, be surprised to find them in a very odd place or a place you'd already searched with no apparent explanation. These types of reality shifts are remarkably commonplace; yet, unless we pay attention to them, they often go unnoticed and unannounced.

HOW ARE QUANTUM JUMPS POSSIBLE?

Consider the idea that many times—possibly even every time—you make a decision or choice, you are actually moving between alternate realities, between parallel worlds. In those alternate realities, there is another possible "you" who you can connect with so strongly that the conscious awareness and energy that is you literally moves into that other reality. When feeling so strongly connected to another self in a different reality, it is possible to gain direct access to the knowledge available only in that time and space and to experience an entirely different self.

What makes quantum jumping possible is that, like a quantum particle, every person has the ability to exhibit quantum behavior. While it may seem extremely improbable that you can do the things quantum particles do—such as tunnel through solid barriers, or make quantum jumps to other alternate times and places—our current understanding of physics suggests such things are within the realm of possibility and can be expected to occur.

Experimental observations at the quantum level change our assumptions about reality as we see that: quantum particles are not always particles and sometimes exist as pure energy; some kind of invisible connection exists between entangled quantum particles, so they move together simultaneously with non-local spooky action at a distance; simply by observing an experiment we are affecting it; and, unlike classical physics, quantum behavior can only ever be predicted by probabilities.

In order to explain some of this truly strange quantum behavior, Niels Bohr theorized that quantum particles exist as waves that might be anywhere until the wave function is collapsed. Hugh Everett III theorized that we exist in a multiverse consisting of many worlds of parallel realities.

Physicist John Cramer theorizes it is possible for information to be exchanged between past and future through a kind of handshake between two points in space-time. Scientists David Bohm and Karl Pribram proposed the universe is a giant hologram, containing matter and consciousness in a single field.

What all this means to someone experiencing a quantum jump is that they can enter another parallel reality by relaxing and imagining they are accessing some kind of bridge, window, or doorway to another world with another self who has another set of characteristics, qualities, or skills. With quantum jumping, one makes the leap from simply imagining oneself in an alternate reality to actually being that other self. In this fashion, a mother who'd moments earlier stood atop a huge boulder holding her child's hand as an enormous tornado raced their way can switch from not being able to imagine herself jumping straight down off a boulder to making that ten-foot leap to safety.

The success of most all visualization methods, affirmations, faking it 'til you make it, the placebo effect, and even simply getting out of bed when you don't feel like it can be attributed to quantum jumping.

WHY DO QUANTUM JUMPS OCCUR?

In order to understand quantum jumps, it's essential that we fully appreciate what "quantum" means. The word "quantum" in the field of physics is defined in the Oxford dictionary as being: "a discrete quantity of energy proportional in magnitude to the frequency of the radiation it represents." "Quantum mechanics" is defined as: "the branch of mechanics that deals with the mathematical description of the motion and interaction of subatomic particles, incorporating the concepts of quantization of energy, wave-particle duality, the uncertainty principle, and the correspondence principle." The whole reason this field of physics studying the very small sprang up in the first place was in pursuit of the true nature of reality. "What is the true nature of reality?" has been the guiding question inspiring generations of physicists to pursue ever smaller particles on the quest to find the most fundamental irre-

Unlike classical physics, quantum behavior can only ever be predicted by probabilities.

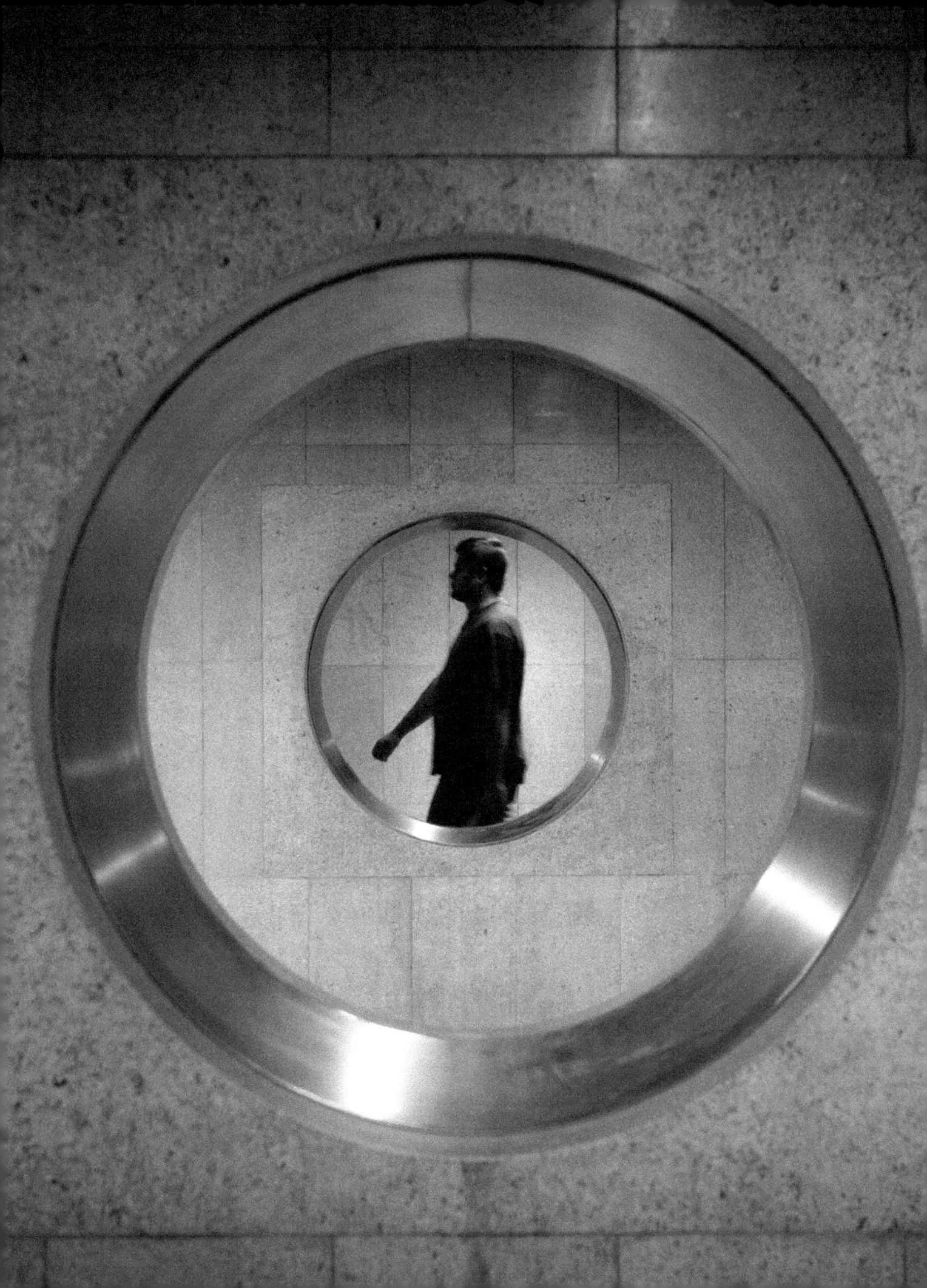

ducible building block from which all that we see and know to be real springs forth. Atoms were found to consist of protons, neutrons and electrons—spinning so rapidly through mostly wide open spaces while invisible to the human eye—yet we know they exist, thanks to experiments with "atom35 smashers." Early discoveries of even smaller bits of matter rocked the world in the twentieth century. But the most unsettling thing to scientists wasn't so much the miniscule size of these quantum particles as it was the way these quantum particles behave.

QUANTUM WEIRDNESS ON THE MACRO SCALE

There are many types of behaviors exhibited at the quantum level that we don't expect to see on the macro scale of our daily lives, mostly because we're unaware of being readily able to observe them with our ordinary senses. Our perception of our world in this new Quantum Age is about to undergo something on par with the Copernican Revolution. In the Copernican Revolution of the sixteenth century, most people worldwide changed their mental model of our solar system from envisioning the sun and planets revolving around the Earth to realizing the Earth revolves around the sun. This changing worldview depends on scientific observations of quantum behavior on the macroscopic scale of physical objects we can readily observe with our ordinary senses. Such aspects of quantum weirdness include: quantum superposition of states, quantum coherence, quantum entanglement, quantum tunneling, and quantum teleportation.

QUANTUM SUPERPOSITION OF STATES

Quantum superposition is a fundamental principle in quantum mechanics by which all possibilities for something in material form exist simultaneously in all possible particular states (or all possible configurations of its properties)—but whenever measured or observed, the result corresponds to only one of those possible states or configurations.

QUANTUM COHERENCE

Quantum coherence is another basic principle in quantum mechanics by which, in any given quantum system, all parts of that system remain in perfect synchronization with one another. There is currently no observable mechanism by which a given quantum system achieves such a state, yet this feature of coherence allows quantum systems to achieve amazing levels of efficiency.

QUANTUM ENTANGLEMENT

Physicist Erwin Schrödinger introduced entanglement as a correlation of different measurement outcomes with the German word *tg*, stating, "Maximal knowledge of a whole system does not necessarily include knowledge of all of its parts, even if these are totally divided from each other and do not influence each other at the present time." There is a level of interconnectedness by which quantum particles move in simultaneous synchronization, even when separated by distance in space.

QUANTUM TUNNELING

Quantum tunneling is a quantum mechanical effect in which particles have a finite probability of crossing an energy barrier, such as the energy needed to break a bond with another particle, even when that quantum particle's energy is less than the energy barrier. Because matter is both particle and waves, something can exist on one side of a barrier, then exist in energy wave form, and then be observed on the other side of a barrier.

QUANTUM TUNNELING

Quantum teleportation is a term used to describe the instantaneous transference of properties from one quantum system to another without physical contact. As for what causes such remarkable behavior at the quantum level of reality—nobody really knows for

All possibilities for something in material form exist simultaneously in all possible particular states.

There is a level of interconnectedness by which quantum particles move in simultaneous synchronization.

sure. The mathematical equations describing quantum behavior work beautifully well, yet the behind-the-scenes why and how of it are anything but obvious. There are numerous physics theories that each explain what's going on in their own unique ways, and these theories are known as 'interpretations' since they provide us with possible explanations for what might be going on, based on sound assumptions. Chief among these theories, which seem to do an excellent job of accounting for "quantum weirdness" are: John Cramer's Transactional Interpretation, Hugh Everett III's Many Worlds Interpretation (MWI), David Bohm's Holographic Interpretation, Leonard Susskind and Raphael Bousso's Holographic Multiverse Interpretation, and Niels Bohr's Copenhagen Interpretation.

JOHN CRAMER'S TRANSACTIONAL INTERPRETATION
Handshake between future and past

John Cramer's transactional interpretation of quantum physics suggests that "handshakes" take place between quantum particles in different points in time and space. In Cramer's interpretation, a particle here and now on Earth instantaneously communicates with particles light-years away in time and space, as one particle sends an "offer" wave and another responds with a "confirmation" wave.

HUGH EVERETT III'S MANY WORLDS INTERPRETATION (MWI)
Many parallel worlds

In the 1950s, Hugh Everett III proposed that every possibility inherent in each wave function is real, and that *all* of them occur. Possibilities become actualities with each measurement that is made, and infinite slightly different realities come into existence as each quantum event is observed. All possibilities are equally real in the multiverse. Parallel universes coexist side-by-side, undetected by one another.

DAVID BOHM'S HOLOGRAPHIC INTERPRETATION
Enfolded order

University of London physicist David Bohm and Stanford University neurophysiologist Karl Pribram proposed that the universe may be like a giant hologram, containing both matter and consciousness as a single field. This model suggests that the objective world "out there" is a vast ocean of waves and frequencies, which appears solid to us because our brains convert that enfolded hologram into unfolded physical material we can perceive with our senses. As the English poet William Blake explains, we thus "... see a world in a grain of sand."

NIELS BOHR'S COPENHAGEN INTERPRETATION
Popping the 'quiff'—collapsing the wave function

The Copenhagen Interpretation of quantum physics was first described and presented by Niels Bohr in Italy in 1927. Bohr suggested that quantum particles exist as waves, which might be anywhere until the wave function is collapsed. As long as nobody looks, each quantum particle is equally distributed in a series of overlapping probability waves, in a superposition of states. An observer is required to assist in ensuring quantum choices are made.

HOLOGRAPHIC MULTIVERSE INTERPRETATION
Many unified parallel worlds

Stanford physicist Leonard Susskind and UC Berkeley's Raphael Bousso assert that the global multiverse is a representation of the many worlds within a single holographic superstructure providing enclosed universes with boundaries. All the physics of the multiverse is encoded upon the boundary in time of the surrounding superstructure, where time is set to infinity. Observers are aware of their own slices of reality in space and time within their respective universes.

INTERPRETING QUANTUM JUMPS

It's important to note that all the above possible explanations for what's happening on the quantum level end with the word "interpretation," reminding us that no physicist yet lays claim to anything akin to a quantum "law" of physics.

The best that's so far been achieved are some beautiful possible topographies and elegant mathematical descriptions. It is clear that John Cramer's Transactional Interpretation of quantum mechanics offers some uniquely helpful insights to assist anyone desiring a quantum jump, as does the relatively new Holographic Multiverse Interpretation. I love the idea that quantum theories can be combined to create imaginative new interpretations in much the same way that chefs create exotically delicious concoctions such as Thai-flavored Mexican burritos!

It's entirely possible that rather than just one of the above interpretations being correct and all others incorrect, several theories may be working together. The Holographic Multiverse Interpretation, for example, is a combination of the Holographic Interpretation with the Many Worlds Interpretation that provides a more holistic, integrated version of many possible worlds. Within a holographic multiverse, there is an interconnectedness between each part of any given parallel universe and all other possible parallel worlds within that holographic multiverse. When the Holographic Multiverse Interpretation is combined with the Transactional Interpretation, we gain an extraordinary view of reality that can truly broaden our minds.

The Transactional Interpretation involves absorption and emission of waves, with perfect symmetry occurring between emitted and absorbed waves. In essence, what is hap-

pening is a synchronized behind-the-scenes choreography in which one point in space-time communicates with another in something akin to a handshake. When you realize that some information is moving forward in time and some backward through time, there is equal significance to receiving information as there is to sending it—both are equally active and involved. As physicist Ruth Kastner points out, "Why should Nature care whether we 'observe' or not...?

The only way that Nature could know or care would be because something physical really happens in such "observations," and the only possible physical process accompanying an "observation" is absorption."

HOW DO QUANTUM JUMPS WORK?

You've probably heard of self-fulfilling prophecies in which people often experience that which they expect. Professional athletes take advantage of this phenomenon by practicing visualization of perfect performance in order to get the best results.

Starting with an understanding that everything is made up of quantum material at its very core, the idea behind quantum jumps is that it's possible to jump to an alternate reality in much the same way that an electron dematerializes at one orbital level and reappears at another. The fundamental principles behind quantum jumping are based upon the behavior of the very smallest particles known in physics—quantum particles. There is a superposition of states in the time of dematerialization in which a quantum particle is between states and is behaving like pure energy rather than like a particular piece of matter. Just as electrons can make energetic leaps from one energetic level to another, people can quantum jump through alternate realities to experience dramatic shifts in physical reality. Quantum jumps can be envisioned as occurring in a multiverse of many alternate realities. Within each one of these realities exists another possible "you" that you can

The universe may be like a giant hologram, containing both matter and consciousness as a single field.

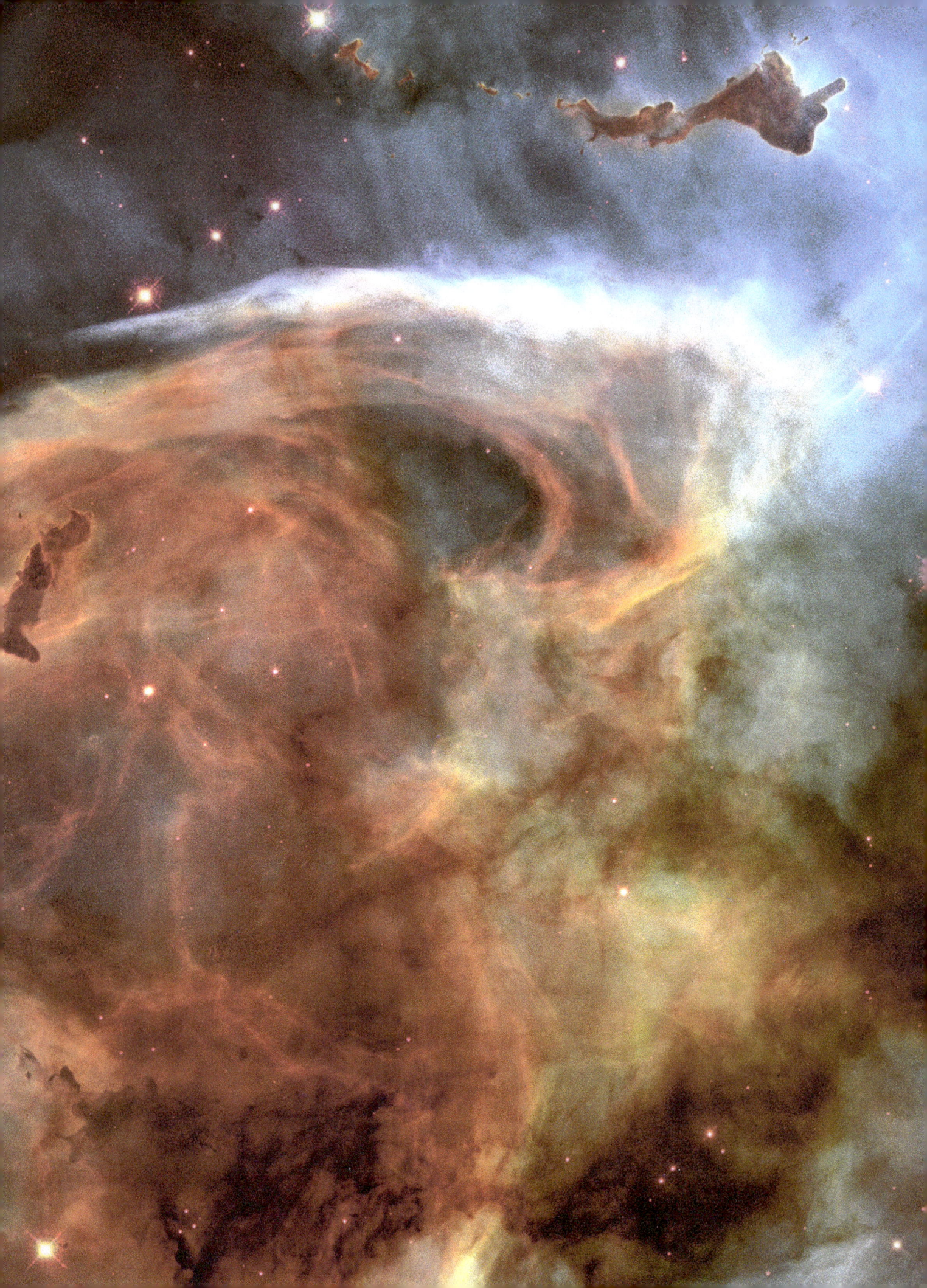

just as easily be.

Anyone who can relax, clear their mind, and envision being different in some way—such as more successful, funny, healthy, wealthy, or wise—can quantum jump. To initiate a quantum jump requires keeping an open mind that you can experience another reality. It is important that you are able to sincerely desire and feel a connection to another reality, envisioning some way of making a connection with it through a bridge, a door, a window or a handshake.

Your ability to form a strong intention, to concentrate, and to get and stay focused while feeling detached from concerns of daily life—relaxed, open-minded, and emotionally energized—are essential. Just as when you shift gears on your car you must first disengage from one gear before re-engaging in a new gear, you must attain a mindset of detachment in order to release connections to physical realities you have felt locked into with your thoughts and feelings. Detachment and disengagement give you a necessary break from identifying as who you've thought you are, so you can experience the ecstasy of feeling relaxed and energized in a state of pure consciousness for a little while. In such a state of pure consciousness, you become aware that you are capable of sensing all possible realities, and you realize that you can emerge from this meditation or lucid dream into the best possible reality for you.

YOU CAN JUMP IF YOU WANT TO

If you can walk, you can dance—and you can quantum jump. Your body is designed for quantum jumping, so learning how to improve your skills can be every bit as simple as making the transition from walking to dancing. The essential spirit of quantum jumping might be summed up in American psychologist William James' words, "If you want a quality, act as if you already have it." Sounds simple enough, right? Well, as you might have suspected, sometimes there can be a little more to it than that. If we were perfectly now-centric beings, with no worries for the future or regrets and misgivings about the past, quantum jumping would be much easier for the simple reason that we'd all be experiencing the benefits of having beginner's mind. The challenges of jumping to a new reality become clear when we start doubting ourselves based on who we think we are based on what we've already done and what we think we can do. These areas are outside the realm of the eternal now, yet most people who don't practice mindfulness tend to worry a fair bit about the future and the past. When we're not mindful, it's easy to get caught up in drama triangles in which we feel like we've been victimized, or like there is a "bad guy," or that we need to rescue someone. What we need, in other words, is the ability to focus exclusively on who we'd most like to be and what we most need to be doing without getting caught up in all the drama we're so used to in our everyday lives. Here's where we can gain some insight from those who study the nature of reality and consciousness in the fields of neuroscience and physics.

Neuroscientist Gregor Thut of the Institute of Neuroscience and Psychology observes, "Despite experiencing the world as a continuum, we do not sample our world continuously but in discrete snapshots determined by the cycles of brain rhythms." Quantum jumping takes advantage of these usually unseen discontinuities, so we can make a leap from one reality to another as smoothly as walking through the one we're already in. And one of the more interesting aspects of quantum jumping is that in addition to making a leap to a parallel reality, we're making changes to our futures and our pasts. You've felt such changes happen to your future and your past any time you've felt increased hope for your future or gratitude for your past... as doubts, worries, regrets, and fears slipped away. As H.G. Wells said in the movie *The Time Machine*, "We all have our time machines, don't we. Those that take us back are

> Just as electrons can make energetic leaps from one energetic level to another, people can quantum jump through alternate realities.

> You can think of what's happening as a large number of possible realities co-existing in a blur of energy waves at every decision point.

memories... and those that carry us forward are dreams." But what if making a leap to a better reality could be easy?

What if we could get help to stay balanced and take our first steps in a new direction when we need it? When we consider the Transactional Interpretation of quantum physics where there's a "handshake" between a possible future point in space-time and now, we see something amazingly special going on.

There is every bit as much involvement from the future point in space-time reaching back to you as there is from you reaching forward for that "brass ring." Why is imagining a future You that is reaching back and giving you a hand up so important?

Because it makes the study of quantum jumps so much easier. You don't need to make such a huge effort. It's just as important to relax, raise your confidence and Qi (internal energy) to a level where you feel closely aligned with your desired future reality.

In June 2006, dozens of scholars traveled from all around the world to gather in San Diego, California, at the "Frontiers of Time: Retrocausation—Experiment and Theory" physics symposium. This very special section of the 87th annual meeting of the Pacific Division of the American Association for the Advancement of Science (AAAS) was convened for the purpose of examining the nature of time... and causality.

Conference organizer and University of San Diego physicist Daniel Sheehan explains, "To say that it's impossible for the future to influence the past is to deny half of the predictions of the laws of physics." Despite the fact that no clear consensus viewpoint yet exists amongst leading researchers in the field of reverse causation (also known as backward causation or retro-causation) as to just how, exactly, the future can influence the past, most physicists do accept the idea of time symmetry. "The tendency is to ignore it, to say it's just a fact of nature that time moves one way," said physicist Michael Ibison from the University of Texas at Austin.

Daniel Sheehan agrees, "People know how to calculate with quantum mechanics, but that's not to say they know what it means. Quantum mechanics is like poetry. The poem is right there, for everyone to see, but it has many different interpretations." While University of Washington physicist John Cramer awaits positive results from his experiment to detect photons of light before they've been emitted, the best current evidence for reverse causation comes from the field of parapsychology, where experiments are being conducted to investigate such things as telepathy, clairvoyance, precognition, psychokinesis, and other types of psi phenomena. While growing numbers of studies in the field of parapsychology, such as those by UC Berkeley physicist Henry Stapp, indicate experimental participants are able to influence radioactive decay of isotopes in the past, few mainstream research laboratories are repeating these experiments.

"You'd think people would want to either refute or confirm some of these reports," said Stapp, "but the only people willing to test them are people who already tend to believe them. Most mainstream labs shy away for fear of sullying their reputations, as if they would be dirtying their hands by even imagining some of this is possible."

Who are our quantum jumping experts? We can look to our top athletes, medical miracle people who've experienced spontaneous remissions of otherwise incurable medical conditions, and our top businessmen and women. We can also learn from survivors who've experienced life-saving miracles; heroes who have acted courageously by "just doing what needed to be done;" people who've had near-death experiences (NDEs); experienced meditators; and people who've worked with lucid dreams, daydreams, and hypnosis to access other realities.

If you've sometimes recalled alternate histories—something like a different ending to a book or movie, or perhaps you've been surprised to hear recent news about a certain celebrity when you clearly remember seeing reports of their death—then you have already quantum jumped.

One of the important keys to success is knowing that there is much more than just one universe. There are many more than just two realities. You can think of what's happening as a large number of possible realities co-existing in a blur of energy waves at every decision point. Amidst all these possible realities, there are some realities you are much more likely to find enjoyable and meaningful.

THREE STEPS TO QUANTUM JUMPS

The following three steps to achieving quantum jumps are meditative in nature, so they tend to work best either while in quiet contemplation or in a daydreamy or hypnotic state. If you have access to a recording device and earphones, you can create your own guided journey through the three steps, playing it back as you fall asleep each night or during a peaceful time of day when you can close your eyes and completely relax.

People who experience miracles are described in Carolyn Miller's book as creating the right conditions for miracles by attaining a detached and peaceful altered state, expecting a positive rather than a negative outcome, and focusing on love rather than fear with a changed perception of what had been viewed as the problem. Carolyn Miller defines a miracle as: "...an instance in which a supernatural power interferes in the natural world," which sounds a lot like quantum jumps or reality shifts to me. As it turns out, the three steps of miracle-mindedness are similar to the three steps for successful quantum jumps.

QUANTUM JUMPING STEPS

1. Attain a relaxed, detached, and peaceful altered state.

2. Feel energized about your visualized posi-

tive outcome.

3. Take positive action in keeping with your new reality.

STEP ONE: ATTAIN A DETACHED, PEACEFUL STATE OF MIND

While you might think of achieving goals in terms of being active and doing things, one surprising truth about quantum jumps is that despite the name, "quantum jump," there's not so much action involved in the jumping as one might think. The required state before making a leap to another reality is more like being in-between states—in the midst of a nice daydream—than making a big effort or exertion. You can access such a detached state of mind through meditation or lucid dreaming.

This sense of peaceful detachment is vitally important because this state of mind allows us to let go of the conscious, ego-driven mindset that got us into whatever challenging situations we are presently engaged. We must let go of what we think is best and believe should occur, so we can maintain a neutral, receptive state of mind. The energy of charged emotions tends to lock realities and particular histories in place—so it's essential that we attain a state of emotional and energetic detachment that allows us to calmly respond to whatever comes next.

We can experience mindful harmonious balance when we appreciate our many possible pasts and futures with gratitude and love rather than regrets and fears. Meditating at such a point of emotional balance and detachment helps us naturally achieve internal attitudinal adjustments, which in turn help us make better choices that we won't regret later on.

The key to meditation is mindful awareness. There are many ways to attain a detached, peaceful state of mind in meditation, including: walking meditation, breathing meditation, silent meditation, chanting meditation, meditating while gardening,

> We must let go of what we think is best and believe should occur, so we can maintain a neutral, receptive state of mind.

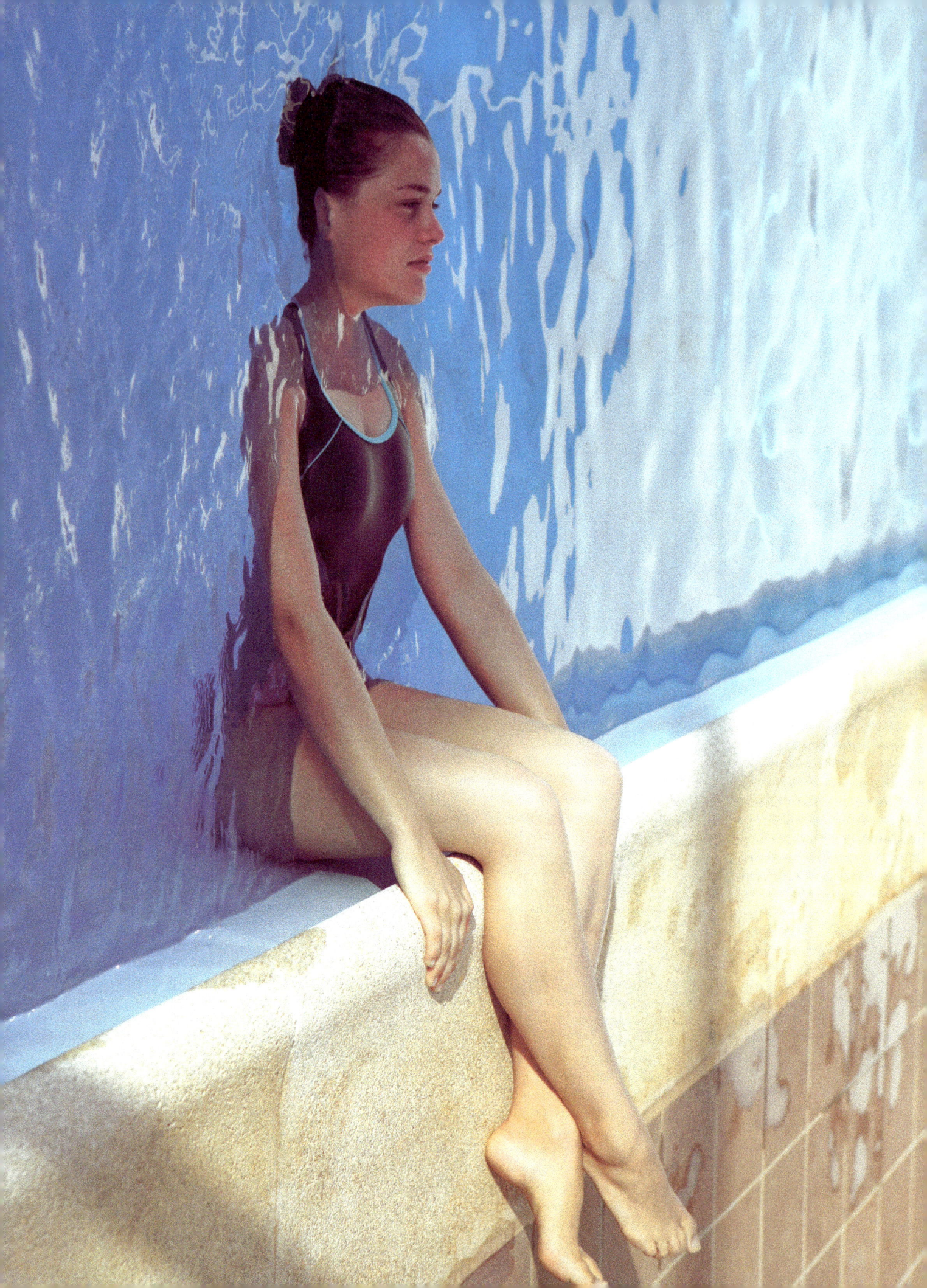

meditating while bathing, or meditating doing dishes or chores.

Just as Asian cultures respect the complementary dynamics of Yin (feminine) and Yang (masculine), the first step in quantum jumping can be thought of as a meditative Zen-like acceptance of all that is while internally "going to our happy place." This is a Yin quality of receptivity that appears to be the opposite of action. If you are experiencing the multiverse like a quantum particle, this state of detached receptivity feels like letting go of your material nature so you no longer fixate on any given point in space-time, and instead spread yourself out in the form of pure energy waves across all possible realities. In such a state of being pure energy, you can envision all possible futures and pasts and quickly see where each choice ends up.

Can you imagine that you and everything and everyone around you exists in a superposition of states? When we achieve a peaceful, detached state of mind, it's analogous to the kind of superposition of all possibilities that a majority of physicists agreed is true for everything—not just tiny quantum particles.

It is possible to contemplate that we can make the best decisions when remembering that, in a multiverse of many possible worlds, everything can happen—and actually is happening—somewhere. In order to arrive at a preferred reality, we must first disengage and detach from our daily struggles by taking a meditative break in the peaceful feeling of calm we experience at the center of all options.

Quantum jumping is very much like shifting gears. When we change gears while driving a car with a stick shift, we move out of one particular reality—such as first gear—by first deselecting all gears as we put our foot on the clutch pedal.

From that place of accessing all possibilities, we can move to the next reality we select—such as second gear. Being conscious of existing in such a superposition of states is akin to being in a state of timelessness... a feeling of being detached from, rather than attached to, everyday reality. From meditating or dreaming in such a timeless place of pure energetic being, we can calmly focus on exactly what we'd most prefer to happen next before returning to our regular mindset and our preferred reality.

STEP TWO:
FEEL ENERGIZED ABOUT THE VISUALIZED OUTCOME

Studies confirm that athletes perform considerably better after first visualizing success. More specifically, the top athletes depend on mental practice or imagery rehearsal of doing what it takes to be their best in order to help guarantee their winning edge. When athletes first practice their maneuvers in their imagination before actual physical performances, studies consistently show they benefit from improvements in skill, confidence, and a sense of calm.

Sports psychologists help Olympic athletes ensure better visualization of success by providing guided visualizations. Such a coach helps ensure that athletes spend 20 minutes or so relaxing first, before beginning mental practice, because they know that best results come from a place of peaceful, relaxed detachment before doing imagery rehearsal. Sports psychologists assist athletes in focusing on visualizing themselves doing better at particular physical activities they've been challenged with before, such as improving a golf swing.

Thanks to magnetic resonance imaging (MRI) scans, neuroscientists have begun to explain a mechanism to account for why imaginary practice can be so extraordinarily effective.

Dr. Thomas Newmark explains, "Internal visualization of specific movements creates neural patterns in the brain, improving neuromuscular coordination. Because the brain tells the muscles how to move, stronger neural patterns thus result in clearer, stronger movement. Results are then reinforced

Being conscious of existing in such a superposition of states is akin to being in a state of timelessness...

Internal visualization of specific movements creates neural patterns in the brain.

by gains made in actual practice, where real muscle activity occurs." While MRI scans can help provide us with rational explanations for the way our muscles respond during imaginary practice, they don't entirely account for all types of improvement athletes enjoy. For example, some visualization suggestions mysteriously appear to work despite there being no precise set of muscle groups the athlete can practice working together.

A couple of case study examples provided in Dr. Newmark's research include the effective suggestion that a golfer drive the ball with "laser-like accuracy" and the beneficial intimation that a football player catch each pass as if "glue keeps the ball stuck" to his hands. Both of these visualizations were effective even though they did not correspond to an obvious set of muscular movements. Clearly there is something more going on than simply programming various muscle groups... something we haven't yet found a way to measure with modern day MRI technology, but that we can achieve through visualization.

Picture yourself moving through your new daily activities in your most desired life. Imagine your future self is reaching a hand out and back to help make it easier for you to think, feel, speak, and behave more in accordance with the person you'd most like to become. Notice what is most noticeably different, and pay attention to how you can start behaving more like this possible future self. Even doing the simplest little actions in the direction of living true to your dreams makes a huge difference.

With each newfound pattern of thought, emotional response, speech, and physical action, you are making it easier for you to develop the most optimal behaviors and habits that best correspond with your new life.

STEP THREE:
TAKE POSITIVE ACTION

To experience positive, memorable, meaningful quantum jumps, you must maintain a lucid state of fearlessness and love while taking positive action in keeping with the reality of your dreams. Your feeling of love must be genuine for best results rather than merely doing what has to be done out of obligation, duty, or expectation. Taking some kind of positive action while feeling so much love is akin to having a good attitude in life: doing what needs to be done with a song in your heart and a skip in your step rather than feeling disconnected or disheartened. When you are facing a situation in which you most desire to make a quantum jump, you probably won't initially be feeling anything close to the level of love you'll need to make the leap to a new reality with such a positive state of unified body, heart, and mind.

So how do you focus on love when you're not starting out feeling love, and fake or forced feelings don't count?

Fortunately, it is possible through focusing awareness in prayer or meditation to nurture your feelings of love. You can jumpstart good feelings of love by remembering, for example, how much you love a favorite pet, best friend, child, or sibling.

When you breathe deeply, slowly, and rhythmically while regaining a deep sense of loving connection to something or someone else, you are helping to naturally harmonize your breathing with your heartbeat with your blood pressure.

Attaining such a healthy state of resonance reduces feelings of stress while increasing a general sense of peace and wellbeing.

Once you feel a strong sensation of love—that you might physically feel as warmth in your heart—you can focus your attention on the reality you are choosing for yourself and know what action you can now take that is in keeping with being the new you.

Imagine that this reality is now choosing and coming toward you just as much as you are now choosing and coming to it, so you are now gaining insights and inspiration regarding what you can best think, say, and do.

GETTING STARTED WITH QUANTUM JUMPS

In truth, you've been quantum jumping without realizing that's what you've been doing for quite some time. The difference between quantum jumping when you know you're doing it consists of learning how to move out of current patterns of thoughts and behaviors to new ones that are associated with the reality you are jumping into.

One of the best ways to get a feel for quantum jumping is to recognize practical applications in matters of importance to you as they arise. Two common types of real-life problems quantum jumping is good at resolving include finding lost things and overcoming health problems.

FROM BROKEN LEG TO UNBROKEN LEG

My friend, Susan, took a moonlit walk by herself one night while on a camping trip to Joshua Tree National Park with some friends. Relishing the excitement of jumping from rock to rock as she used to do as a young girl, Susan didn't notice she'd misjudged one jump, until she landed painfully on her right leg.

She felt like her leg was broken and, when she visited the emergency room at the hospital, this news was confirmed by Susan's doctor who told her, "You broke your fibula." Because this hospital was a teaching hospital, a supervising doctor also examined Susan's X-rays and confirmed the first doctor's assessment, saying to Susan, "You've broken your fibular head." At this point, Susan called me and we spoke on the phone about her injury, and we did some energy work on her broken leg to speed healing. I envisioned her leg being healthy with bones strong and unbroken and, at some point during our conversation, Susan told me she felt something like an itchiness where her fibula was broken. I told Susan, "That's a very good sign! Feeling itchiness is often an indication of that part of the body healing."

Later in the week, Susan went to her appointment for a follow-up visit at the clinic. While Susan was waiting, she asked a medic if she could please look at her X-rays while she waited.

He flipped on the viewing lights, granted her permission to see her X-rays, and left the room. Susan pulled two different X-rays out of the envelope and examined them closely. She couldn't see anything that looked like a break, crack, or any other kind of disturbance, but figured to herself, "I'm no doctor, and I'm not trained in reading X-rays. I probably just don't know what I'm looking for."

"When the orthopedic doctor entered the room, she said she'd just looked at my X-rays and didn't understand my diagnosis, since she didn't see a broken bone! She said she even asked the radiologist to look at them, and he didn't see anything either." Susan found it amusing to watch her try to explain how this could happen. At first, it seemed like she was blaming the younger attending physician who'd first told Susan she broke her fibula when she was in the emergency room that Monday. But then, when Susan told her that not only did he look at her X-rays, but also the supervising physician confirmed Susan's leg was broken.

At this point, the doctor became flustered, not wanting to admit hospital error, while clearly confused about what had happened. She fiddled with Susan's leg—poking, twisting, prodding. While Susan flinched a bit, it was more because she was anticipating pain than actually feeling pain. When the doctor asked Susan if anything hurt, Susan told the doctor, "It really only feels like someone is pressing on a bruise you might have received in some random way." The doctor responded, "Well, that's probably what you did. You might have just bruised the bone." Not only was Susan's leg healed, but so were her original X-rays!

After Susan heard this rather startling announcement, she came home to search for her paperwork that had originally been sent

> Even doing the simplest little actions in the direction of living true to your dreams makes a huge difference.

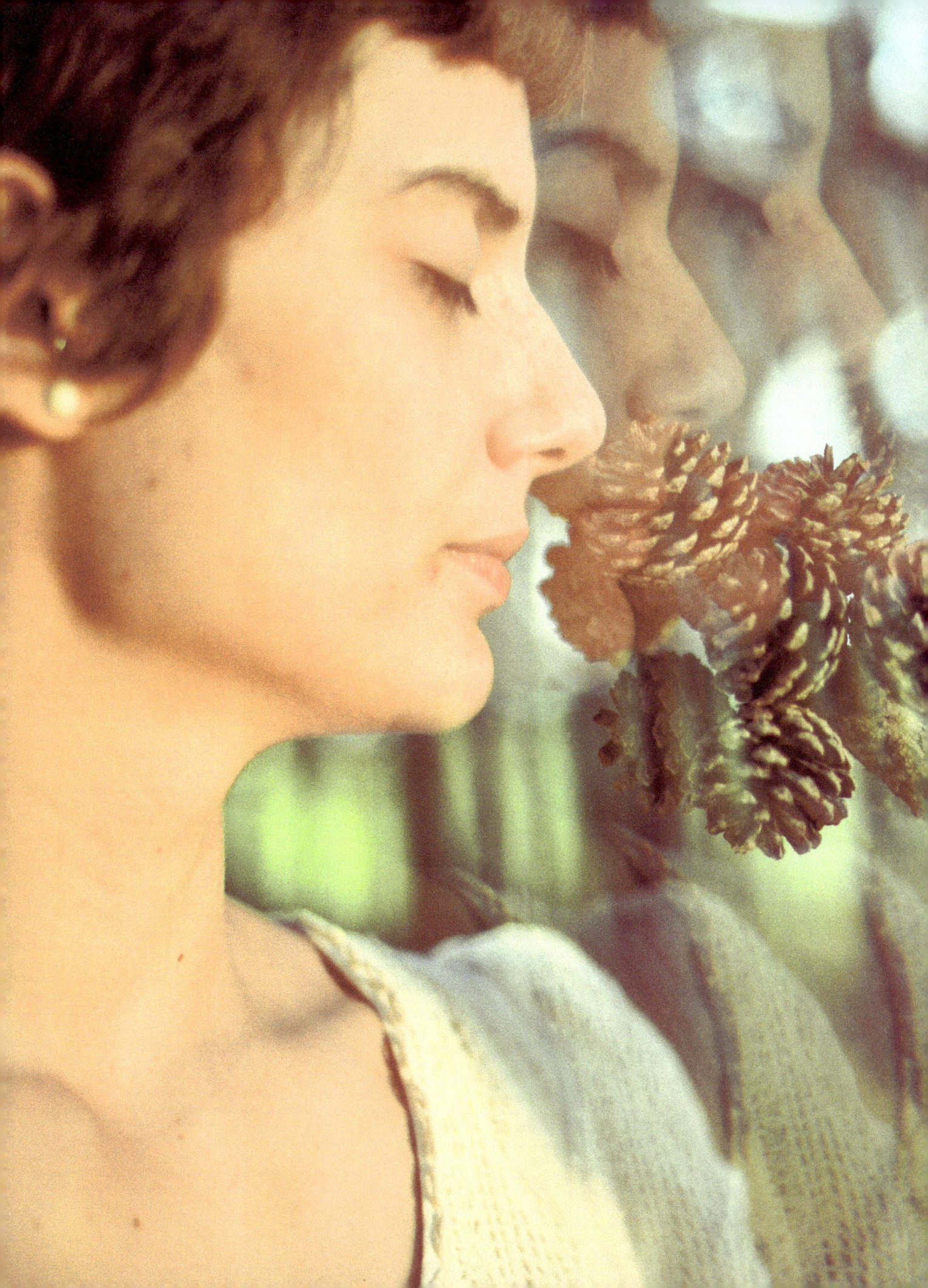

home with her after her initial visit to the hospital. This paperwork was the standard care printout for "a broken extremity;" and Susan recalled that further down there was mention of "a broken fibular head."

Susan told me while searching for the missing documentation, "I need this paperwork to show my employers why I've been missing work and needed to visit the emergency room." Susan's house was hardly a mess of paperwork, and she was quite annoyed to have lost the papers that could prove she hadn't made up the whole thing and taken so many days off work for no reason. A while later, while doing some house cleaning, Susan was surprised to find her missing paperwork...under her television set! She doesn't put anything there—it seemed like it had just suddenly appeared there!

Excerpted with permission from Quantum Jumps: An Extraordinary Science of Happiness and Prosperity by Cynthia Sue Larson.

Cynthia Sue Larson *is a best-selling author and life coach who helps talented people struggling with unsatisfying lives find love, meaning, and prosperity. She has a degree in physics from UC Berkeley, and teaches meditation and martial arts. She has been featured in numerous shows including the History Channel, Coast to Coast AM, and BBC. Endorsed by Dr. Larry Dossey, Fred Alan Wolf, and Stanley Krippner, Cynthia Sue Larson's newest book, Quantum Jumps, describes the science of instantaneous transformation emerging from recent research findings in physics, biology, and psychology. Vist her website: realityshifters.com*

In truth, you've been quantum jumping without realizing that's what you've been doing for quite some time.

Deep Love: The Art of Creating Conscious Relationships

BY GAY & KATHYLN HENDRICKS

Caitlyn came to us at the age of 56. It was a year since the breakup of her second marriage, which had lasted six years. She was still heavyhearted about it.

"Is this the end of the line?" she asked us bluntly. "Should I forget about the whole relationship thing and just settle for what I have.

"Which is?"

"I have a really good life, just with no man in it."

Caitlyn's situation was like that of many single people with whom we've worked. She had a good life going on her own, but she was feeling the ache of something missing from it. She was up against a barrier so significant we call it Barrier Number One.

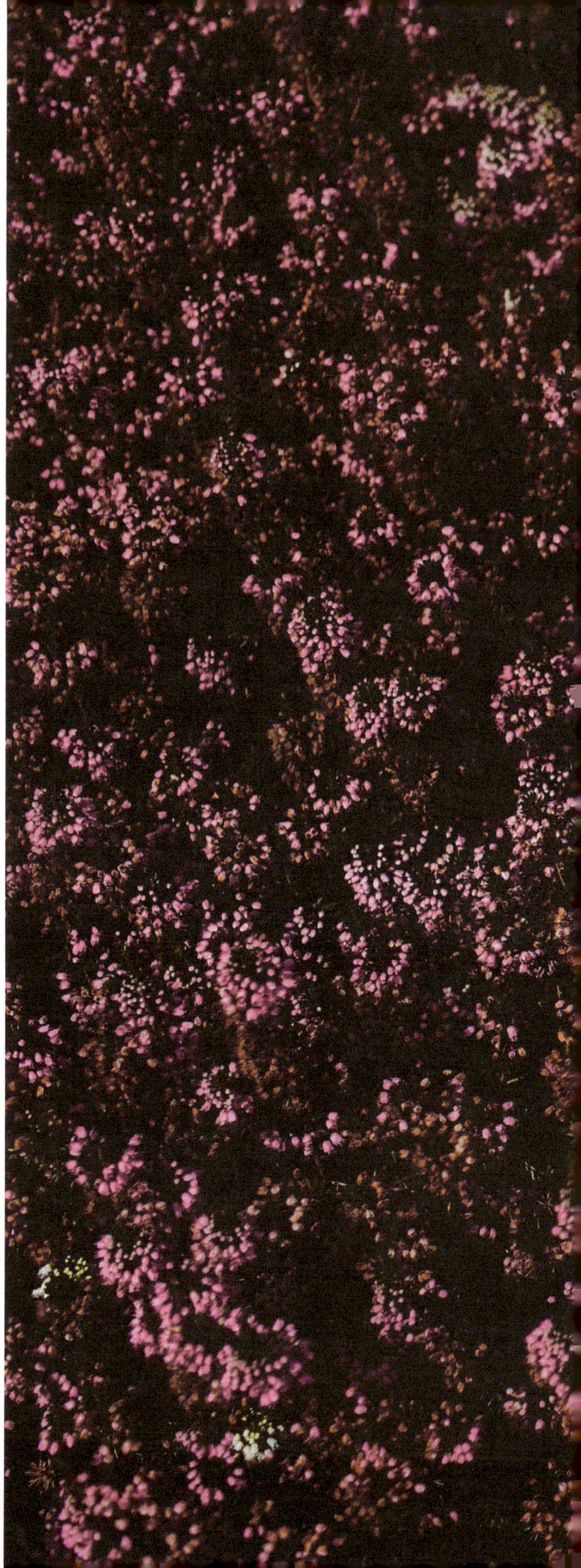

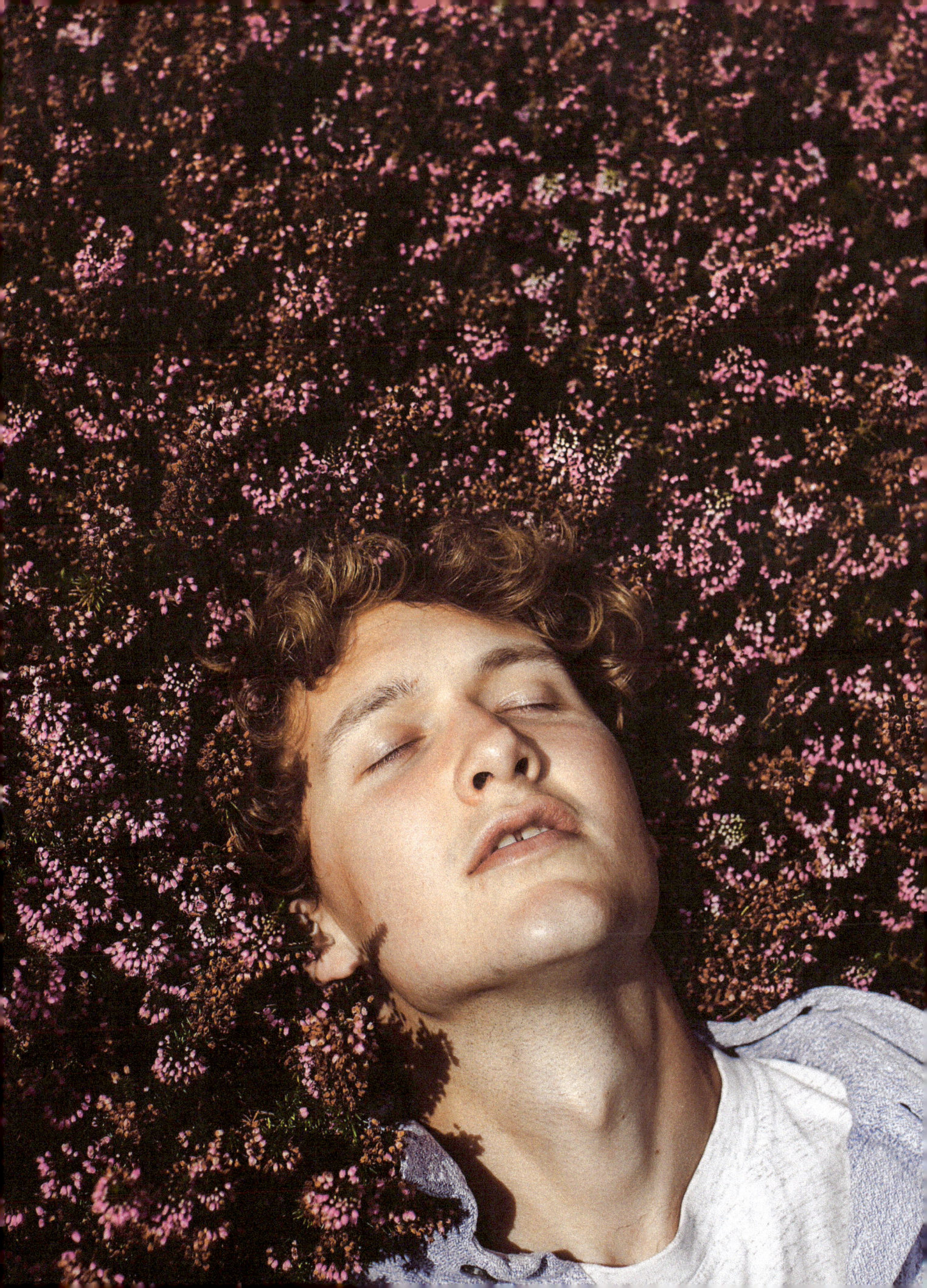

When you send out mixed messages, the most unconscious one is always the one people hear.

Getting Past Barrier Number One: Do You or Don't You?

The first barrier is when you haven't landed on actually wanting a lasting love relationship in your life right now. Part of you does, part of you doesn't. Perhaps without your even realizing it, this internal barrier is keeping you from success in the external quest to create lasting love in your life.

There is a solution to Barrier Number One—a way of clearing it out of the way. Best of all, it won't cost you a cent to get a lifetime supply of it. The solution is a special kind of commitment, a vow you make in the sacred depths of yourself. The power of this commitment releases you from the grip of despair and sends you into the future equipped with a foolproof navigation tool for your journey.

Picture yourself looking into the mirror and speaking a vow to your deepest self, a commitment that goes something like this: *I commit to attracting a loving relationship into my life, a love that lasts and grows over time.*

Making that statement takes you off the bench and onto the field. That's where the action takes place. One big problem we've found is that single people send out mixed messages about whether or not they really want to manifest an intimate relationship. The even bigger problem is that most of them don't realize they're doing it. When you send out mixed messages, the most unconscious one is always the one people hear. For example, if ten minutes into a lunch date you decide you don't really like the person across from you, you're stuck with an unpleasant alternative. You could go radically blunt and say, "I've decided I don't really like you. Let's finish eating by ourselves." Most people, though, opt for a more conventional approach: you go ahead and finish lunch in a polite manner, while pretending your attitude of "I don't really want to be here" isn't there lurking in the background. The trouble with this approach is that attempting to silence or ignore your genuine feelings often

makes the other person perceive them even more loudly and clearly.

A sincere commitment breaks that spell. When you make a sincere vow to your deepest self and the universe around you, something like "I commit to creating the relationship of my dreams in real life," you come off the bench and onto the field.

Getting Through Barrier Number Two: Settling For Less

Don't stop there, though. There's another key commitment you can make to amp up your manifestation power.

Picture yourself again looking into the mirror and making a second sincere vow: *I specifically commit never to settle for less than what I really want.*

This commitment is just as important as the first one; settling for less than what you really want in relationships is a virulent plague in the 21st century. To avoid the plague, you'll not only need to make a sincere vow never to settle for less, you'll also need to do some clear thinking about what you want and don't want.

We spent the better part of a morning working with Caitlyn on these issues. As we heard more of her relationship history, it spelled out a pattern of undervaluing herself, leading to settling for less. She repeatedly put herself in relationships with men that caused her to lose both self-respect and money. What she had put up with—from bankruptcy to drunk-tank bailouts to catching a new husband in bed with the maid of honor—astonished even us.

She also had to face an issue from her past that was causing her to be ambivalent about creating a new relationship. During the whole year since the breakup, she had never simply sat with her grief and felt it consciously. Instead she'd kept herself busy by joining three different singles websites, corresponding with and rejecting "more than a hundred men" on the various sites, and even putting a highly detailed personal ad in the newspaper.

To change the pattern, we first asked Caitlyn to devote a few moments to being with the grief through Full-Spectrum Presencing. "Take a few easy breaths and feel the places in your body where you still feel sad about the breakup." Once she slowed down to honor her authentic feelings for a moment, her mood visibly brightened. She said, "Oh, wait, I think I just made a connection."

At a certain point in each relationship she would start to bottle up feelings out of fear of causing conflict. Invariably, after a while the bottle would pop, leading to noisy conflicts of the sort she feared most. As she explored the issue she realized it was the central drama in her parents' ongoing battle, which led to their divorce when she was five years old. Both her parents would hide their feelings until a blowout occurred every week or two. By the time they divorced, Caitlyn had soaked up so much of the pattern by osmosis that she repeated it unwittingly in her adult relationships.

Getting Over Barrier Number Three: Placing Your Order

Full-Spectrum Presencing opened the gate for Caitlyn, but she also needed to do some "real world" work on attracting a new relationship into her life. In our work with singles, we have found that in order to attract a quality relationship, they need to identify at least three things they want and three things they don't want.

Most people repeat old destructive patterns because they haven't made a clear commitment to something better. At midlife and beyond, the pressure intensifies to break free of these patterns. One common pattern is to know what you don't want but not know what you want. Another common pattern is the opposite: you're clear about what you want but haven't given conscious thought to what you don't want.

So if you're single, check in with yourself. Are you clear on the top three things you want in a close relationship and the top three things you don't want? If so, take a moment to review them right now. If not, get clear right now by asking: *What is the #1 thing that's important for me to have in a lasting love relationship?* Perhaps it's honesty or freedom or a sense of shared beliefs—everyone's #1 is slightly different from others'. What's yours?

Do the same for your #2 and #3 most important things to have in a close relationship. If you've already gotten clear about the three things you most don't want to repeat in your next relationship, review them now.

If not, start by asking: *What is the absolute most important thing I never want to have in a relationship again?* Perhaps it's that you never want to be in a relationship with an addict again, or that you never want to be with someone who doesn't like kids again. Whatever your three biggest "don't want's" are, make a list of them so you're absolutely clear about them.

It's like when you set off on a trip. If you're absolutely clear you want to visit Chicago, Calcutta, and Copenhagen, and you also know for absolute sure you don't want to go to Borneo, Brisbane, and the Bronx, your chances of ending up where you want to be are greatly enhanced.

Sometimes you need to be forceful in stating a "don't want." Certain relationship problems are toxic and need to be avoided, like an allergen. For example, Gay is allergic to sesame seeds and sesame oil, which he learned the hard way from his first trip to a Chinese restaurant when he was a kid. "Now, when I order in a restaurant, I go out of my way to ask if there is sesame involved. I also don't handle MSG or peanut oil well, so I usually ask that they not be used either. I eventually even found a Chinese restaurant that caters to finicky people. The first time I went there, I asked my inevitable question to the waiter. He drew himself up in pride and said, 'Sir, there has never been MSG or sesame oil on our premises.'" We think you should be just that finicky about your love life.

Most people repeat old destructive patterns because they haven't made a clear commitment to something better.

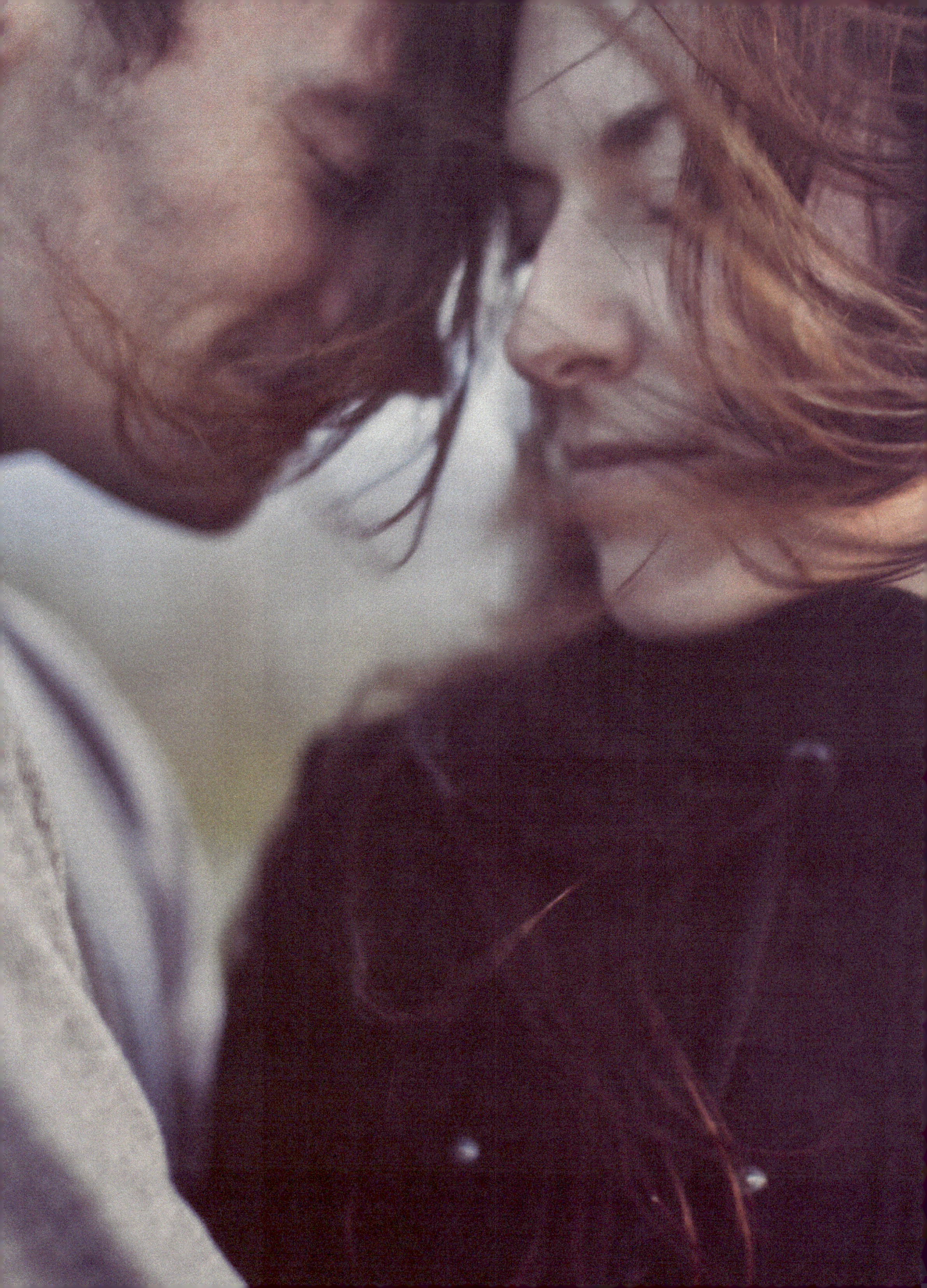

Ordering up a lasting love relationship is like ordering a meal, but with one specific difference; you need to be clear about what you want and don't want. When you order in a restaurant, you don't usually need to list what you don't want, unless you have experienced toxicity in some past relationship with an item. You can just say, "Short stack of blueberry pancakes, two eggs on the side, over medium," as Gay did on a recent visit to Bonnie Lu's Country Café, and with three simple, positive commands you can get the breakfast you want.

Relationships are different, because for relationships to succeed, you need to be really clear about what you don't want. More strongly put, you need to be clear about what you absolutely will not put up with. You might have a list of more than three things fitting that description, but we've found it useful to start with a sturdy foundation of three.

Caitlyn's three positive "wants" were **1.** we have respect and admiration for each other, **2.** we're best friends as well as married to each other, and **3.** we have fun together. In past relationships she'd had glimpses of those qualities but had never put them all together in one relationship.

Caitlyn's three "don't wants" were simple, straightforward, and obviously based on a lot of painful life experience. She didn't want anybody in her life with **1.** financial problems, **2.** addiction issues, or **3.** a history of cheating.

The Ultimate Step

The ultimate step in freeing yourself from the past is also the ultimate step to opening yourself to a new mate in your life. It only takes a split second to take the step, but it has such power that it influences every one you take from then on. It's the moment when you love yourself unconditionally, exactly as you are, for everything you've done and not done. It's the moment when you love yourself for being alone, the forgiving gift to yourself of

For relationships to succeed, you need to be really clear about what you don't want.

Release your urge to want it to be different. Let it be.

celebrating your singularity.

It doesn't matter if you love the unlovable in yourself for ten seconds or a tenth of a second—once you've felt it, even for a moment, you've opened the secret door to creating relationship magic.

Take a moment right now to feel the power of this new state of consciousness we're referring to. First, let go of expectation: if you're single, release the idea that you ought to have a mate. Let go of any other future-facing fantasies you might have about your love life.

Then, let go of whatever has gone on in the past. Everything that happened is beyond your control now. Nothing you can do can change it. The healing move that allows you to go beyond the pain of the past is to accept it fully, as it is. Release your urge to want it to be different. Let it be.

When you free yourself from the future and the past, you are free to innovate now. Your energy is no longer tied up in wanting the past to be different or the future to be any preconceived way. You're in the present, this very moment, an open opportunity to create your new life.

Now all you have to do is add a light intention to this open state of consciousness. A light intention is a gentle aiming of your energy in a certain direction. We call it a "light intention" to distinguish it from a heavy intention such as "I've got to manifest a mate or else my life means nothing." All you need to do is nudge the universe in the direction of sending you the right sort of mate for you. At the same time, let yourself and the universe know that you are going to be just fine without one, that the growing love and respect you have for yourself is big enough to embrace yourself whether you are solo or mated.

This article is an excerpt from Conscious Loving Ever After: How to Create Thriving Relationships at Midlife and Beyond by Gay Hendricks & Kathlyn Hendricks. It is pub-

lished by Hay House (Oct. 2015) and available in bookstores and online at hayhouse. com

Gay Hendricks, Ph.D., *has been a leader in the fields of relationship transformation and body-mind therapies for over 45 years. After earning his Ph.D. in counseling psychology from Stanford, Gay served as professor of Counseling Psychology at the University of Colorado for 21 years. He has written and co-authored (with Katie) 35 books, including the bestseller Conscious Loving, used as a primary text in universities around the world. Gay has offered seminars worldwide and appeared on more than 500 radio and television shows, including Oprah, CNN, CNBC, 48 Hours and others. Visit his website: hendricks.com*

Katie Hendricks, Ph.D., BC-DMT, *is passionate about the power of embodied integrity and emergence and she continuously promotes creative expression in service of a direct experience of life, wholeness and evolutionary collaboration. She has been a pioneer in the field of body-mind integration for over forty years and has an international reputation as a seminar leader, training professionals from many fields in the core skills of conscious living through the lens of body intelligence. Katie earned a Ph.D. in Transpersonal Psychology and is a Board Certified-Dance/Movement Therapist. Visit her website: hendricks.com*

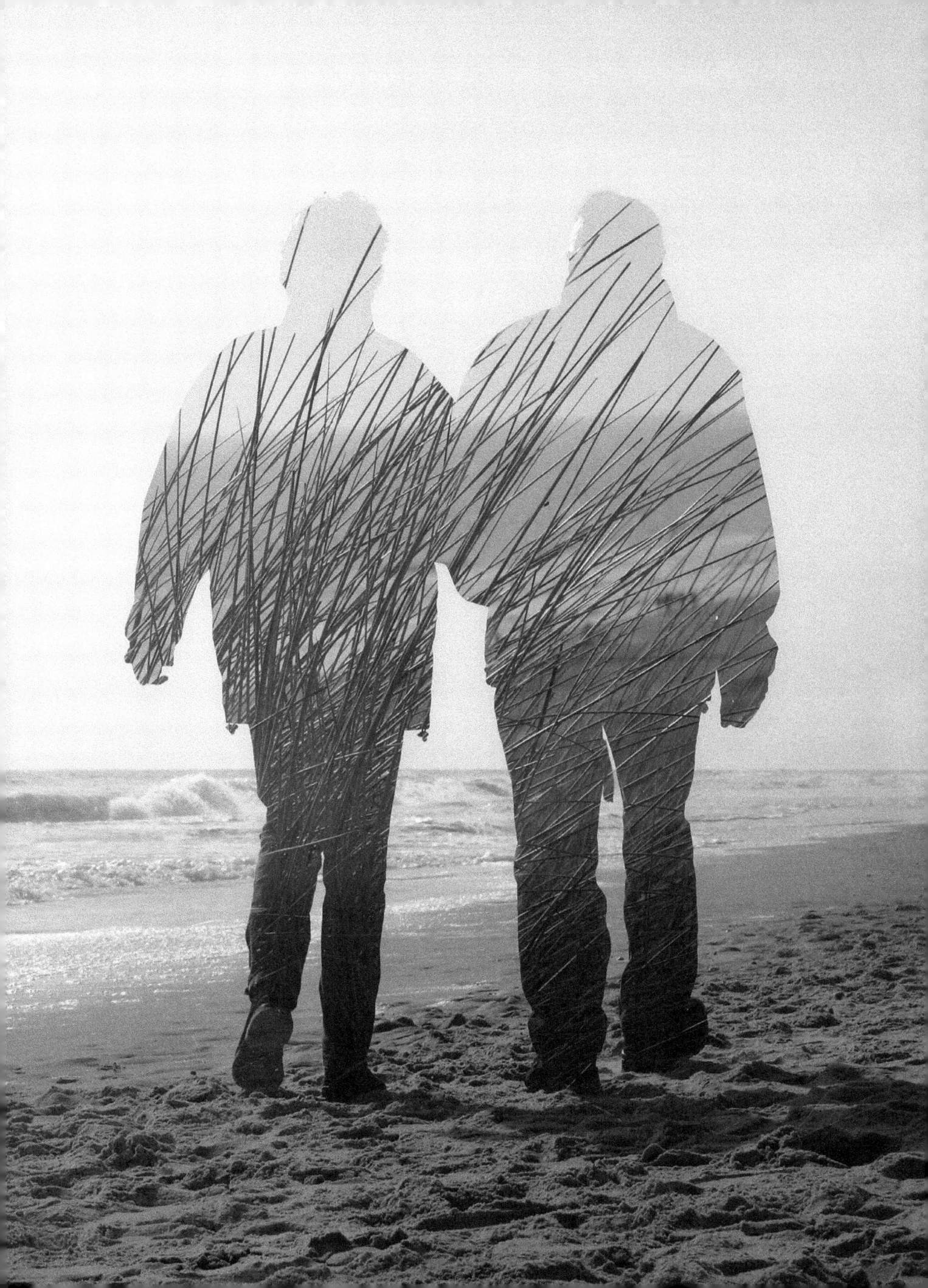

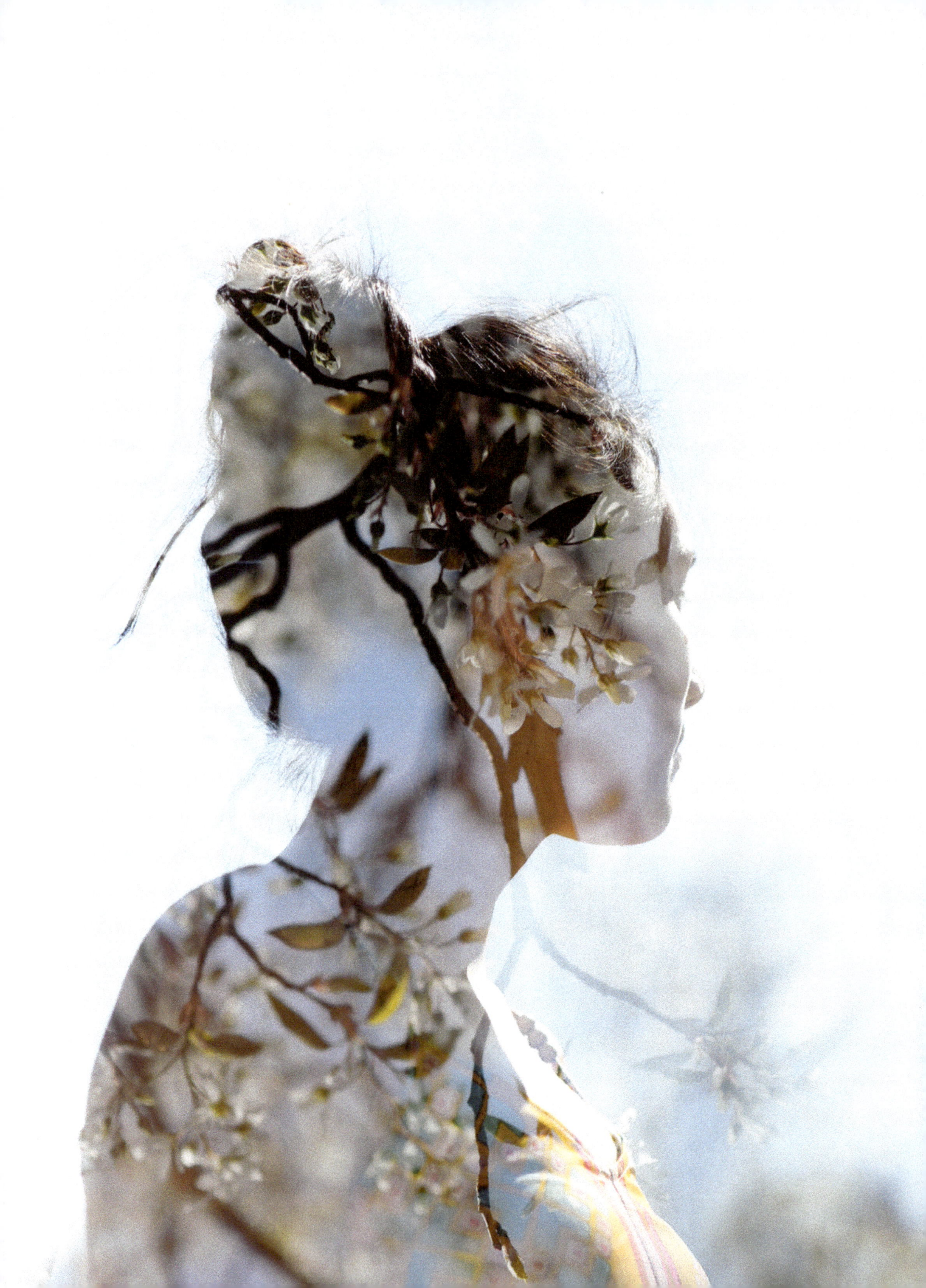

How Nature Changes Your Brain

There's no question that nature soothes the soul, but recent research is also showing that it alters the mind as well

BY JUSTIN FAERMAN

There's no question that immersing your-self in nature is therapeutic on many levels; after all, the process has inspired some of the world's greatest poetry, works of art, and philosophy, from zen koans to the enlightenment thinkers and beyond. However, recent research is now giving some insight into exactly why: it turns out that the simple act of walking or being in nature actually changes the brain in some remarkable ways.

You see, most of us today live in cities and spend far less time outside in green, natural spaces than people did several generations ago; and this fact has encouraged researchers to begin studying the effects this is having on us as inherently biological and nature-dependent creatures. There is a growing body of science-backed evidence that has been accumulating over the last few decades showing a definitive link between exposure to nature, or lack thereof, and altered neurochemistry and psychological states. City dwellers, studies have shown, have been found to have a much higher risk for anxiety, depression, and other mental illnesses than people living outside of urban areas, in more natural and nature-rich settings, or even simply those that live near parks in the same cities. And, in fact, city dwellers who visit natural environments have lower levels of stress hormones immediately afterward than people who have not recently been outside.

But just how a visit to a park or other green space alters our moods has been unclear until recently. Does the act of immersing ourselves in nature actually change our brains in some way that affects our emotional health?

That possibility fascinated Gregory Bratman, a graduate student at the Emmett Interdisciplinary Program in Environment and Resources at Stanford University, who has been studying the psycho-emotional effects of urban living. In a previous study conducted by Bratman, he and his colleagues found that participants who walked, even briefly, through a distinctively lush, green, nature-rich area of the Stanford campus had a marked decrease in anxiety, negative thinking (rumination), were simultaneously more attentive and happier, and had noticeably improved memory afterward than participants who had walked for the same amount of time near heavy traffic.

Inspired by his findings, Bratman and his colleagues then decided to undertake a further study to examine the neurological mechanisms that might underlie the effects of being outside in nature.

The new study, which was recently published in *Proceedings of the National Academy of Sciences*, closely scrutinized what effect time spent in nature would have on a person's tendency to brood, which in the world of cognitive science, essentially means to fall into a pattern of negative thinking and focus. Have you ever fretted over thoughts of what is wrong or "bad," or out of alignment in your life or the world? That's brooding.

It may seem like an interesting choice of states to study; however, brooding is strongly associated with increased activity in a portion of the brain known as the subgenual prefrontal cortex, giving Bratman a definitive brain region to monitor to measure actual changes in neurological functioning. Self-reporting psychological assessments are one thing; brain scans showing actual physical changes in neurological activity are another entirely,

It turns out that the simple act of walking or being in nature actually changes the brain in some remarkable ways.

City dwellers who visit natural environments have lower levels of stress hormones immediately afterward.

free from the subjective bias of self-reporting and hinting at actual underlying mechanisms for the shift in mood and perception.

Bratman and his colleagues gathered 38 healthy, adult city dwellers and had them complete a questionnaire to determine their normal level of brooding, as well as undergo brain scans of the subgenual prefrontal cortex to get a baseline reading to compare with the post-walk scans.

The scientists then randomly assigned one half of the participants to walk alone, without music, for 90 minutes through a quiet, lush, park-like portion of the Stanford campus or next to a loud, hectic, multi-lane highway in Palo Alto at their own pace. Immediately following their walks, participants returned to Bratman's lab and repeated both the questionnaire and the subgenual prefrontal cortex brain scan.

As you might expect, those who walked along the highway did not experience significant changes in their self-reported psychological assessments or their brain scan scores. Blood flow to their subgenual prefrontal cortex, which is a measure of the region's activity, was still high and their brooding scores remained unchanged.

But the participants who had walked through the lush, tree-lined park areas showed meaningful improvements in their mental health, according to their scores on the questionnaire and the activity in their brain scans, which indicated significantly reduced blood flow to the subgenual prefrontal cortex. That portion of their brains was quieter, and they were not dwelling on the negative aspects of their lives as much as they had been before the walk.

These results demonstrate that there is much more than a shift in self- and world-perception going on as we immerse ourselves in nature—our physiology and neurological activity is shifting as well, with changes that echo through the hormonal and neuropeptide cascade in the body and mind. Nature, it turns out, not only soothes the soul, but

makes our journey through life much more peaceful and enjoyable as well—something that many of us inherently knew, but now also understand the physiological mechanics of as well.

Justin Faerman *is a visionary change agent, entrepreneur and healer dedicated to evolving global consciousness, bridging science and spirituality and spreading enlightened ideas on both an individual and societal level. He is the co-founder of Conscious Lifestyle Magazine and a sought after coach and teacher, known for his pioneering work in the area of flow. He is largely focused on applied spirituality, which is translating abstract spiritual concepts and ideas into practical, actionable techniques for creating a deeply fulfilling, prosperous life. Connect with him at artofflowcoaching.com*

WE PLANT A TREE FOR EACH ISSUE YOU RECEIVE

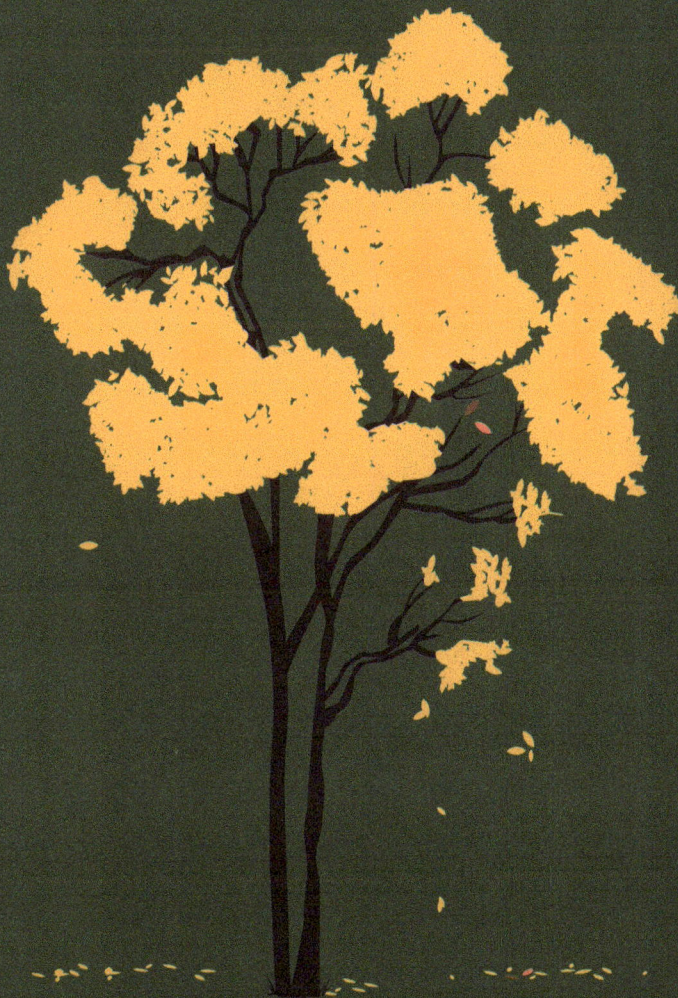

Conscious Lifestyle Magazine is committed to giving back to the planet that gives life to us all. That's why we work closely with *The Eden Projects* to plant a tree in your honor for every issue you receive. The more people who subscribe, the more trees we plant. Together, we create a better world.

The Eden Projects is a 501(c)3 non-profit organization dedicated to planting trees and creating sustainable, meaningful work for local communities in Ethiopia, Madagascar and Haiti. To date, The Eden Projects have planted over **100 million trees worldwide**. Learn more at edenprojects.org.

ConsciousLifestyle
magazine

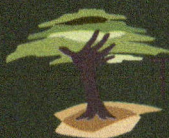

The Eden Projects

Finding Your True Self

*5 Practices for Discovering Your Unique Voice
Through Creative Self-Expression*

By Julia McCutchen

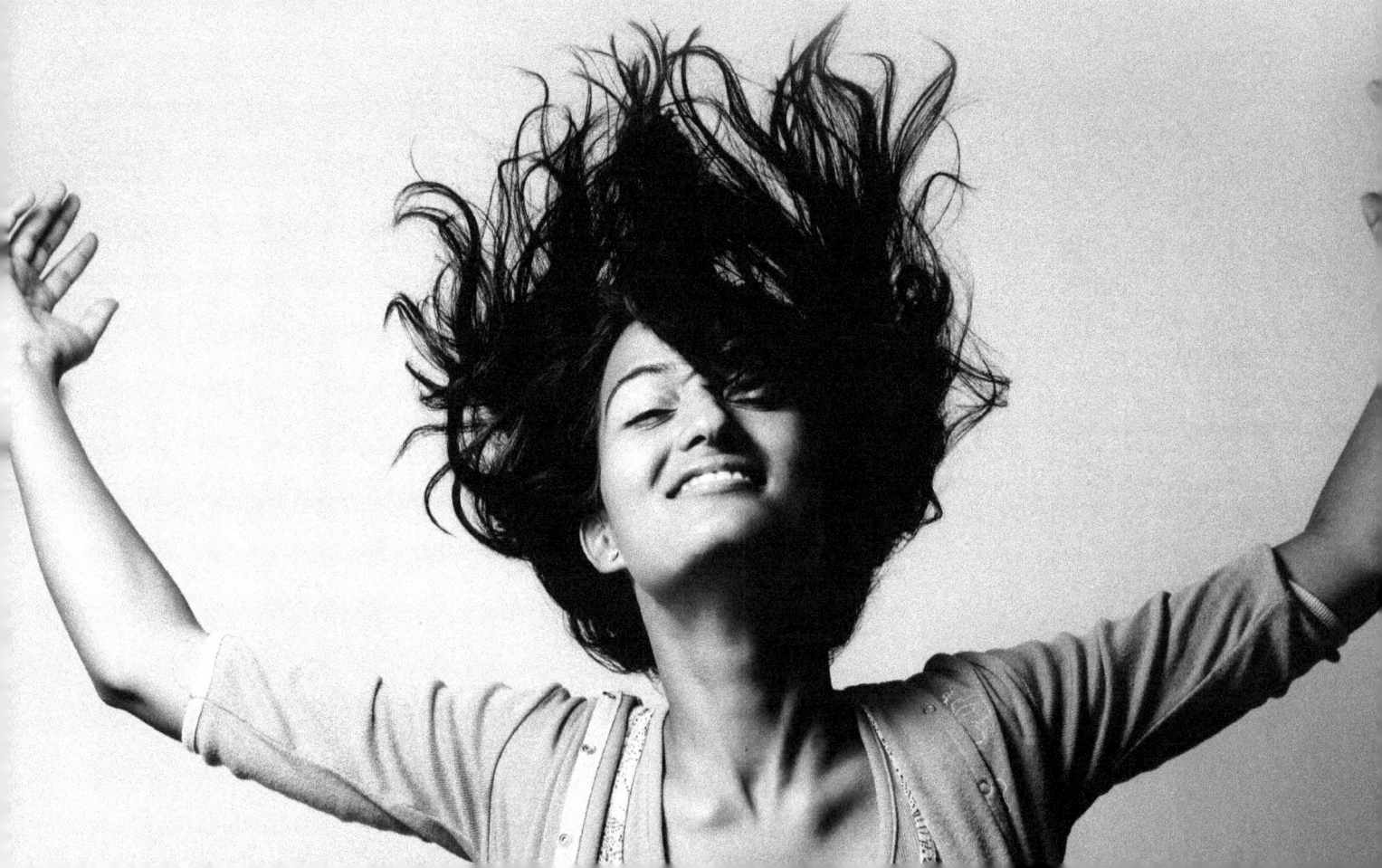

There's a strong inner impulse underlying the dreams that many of us have; it's a yearning to re-connect with who we truly are, discover our true calling, and express ourselves authentically in the world.

When we do, our lives are transformed from what often feels like an uphill struggle into a graceful, conscious and creative flow. Challenges still arise; yet we handle them more skilfully as we accept the reality of what is and show up to take awakened action to share our gifts with purpose and passion.

Yet despite the joy of conscious living, following through on these sometimes subtle but always significant inner impulses is not straightforward.

The reason is that we've mostly been taught how we should be and what we ought to do with our lives. So we strive to fulfill the brief we've been given by our parents, teachers, and other figures of authority; then one day, a major life event stops us in our tracks and we wake up to the realization that we're not feeling happy and fulfilled.

The Shift From Everyday to True Self

Conscious Writing is a holistic and practical approach to creative awakening that teaches us to pay attention to our intuitive impulses and make it a priority to connect with inner truth before taking outer action.

Conscious Writers learn to recognize that the conditioned patterns of thought and behavior that create a life of "should" belong to the everyday self. This is also the source of our anxieties, fears and the inner critic we all have that judges, criticizes, and often holds us back from realizing our full potential.

The shift that Conscious Writing guides us toward is the discovery of our true self and our natural ability to express our true voice, on the page and in the world.

When we expand into the totality of who we already are, we create, write, and live our lives from the eternal part of us that is completely free of conditioning. This leads us to discover our core purpose and make the contribution that only we can make.

Jenny's Story

Jenny was born with a cleft lip and spent a large proportion of her childhood in and out of the hospital undergoing multiple operations to correct her facial disfigurement. The trauma of the physical procedures was compounded by the bullying she received at school and the shame she felt for looking different. Understandably she developed a paralyzing fear of being visible in the world.

During her teenage years she made a significant decision, "If I can't be beautiful, I'll be smart." So she worked hard and excelled at school, continued her studies into further education culminating in a Ph.D., and created the reality of succeeding as an academic.

When Jenny first approached me for guidance, she wanted to learn how to write from her heart to explore the territory beyond intellectual academia. As I introduced her to the principles and practice of Conscious Writing, she gradually opened up to new realms of possibility with her writing.

Simultaneously, she experienced a significant opening within herself as she connected ever more deeply with her true self.

The flowering of Jenny's Conscious Writing transformation began showing up more regularly on the page; not just in the way she was writing but also through the content. She discovered that she felt passionate about spreading the message that we are all essentially born whole, regardless of physical difference.

It took a great deal of courage for Jenny to make the shift from writing privately to sharing her work publicly. However, her commitment to her true calling combined with a Conscious Writing Retreat experience finally enabled her to cross that threshold and launch her "Born Whole" blog.

Jenny is now writing freely from her heart and is developing her new vocation through her writing and as a volunteer for the charity Changing Faces.

> Conscious writing is a holistic and practical approach to creative awakening that teaches us to pay attention to our intuitive impulses.

Discovering your true self and expressing your true voice lead to living an authentic and inspired life.

Discovering Your True Self and Expressing Your True Voice

Even if you don't have any inclination to write, you can still benefit hugely from the principles and practice of Conscious Writing. This is because discovering your true self and expressing your true voice lead to living an authentic and inspired life that is filled with genuine purpose and passion.

So how do we begin?

Conscious Writing trains us to start with inner preparation because the state of consciousness we're in when we do any kind of creative work shapes our experience and the end result. As Conscious Writers, we work with seven core principles that support us to become, and remain, conscious:

1. Presence
2. Alignment
3. Authenticity
4. Balance
5. Simplicity
6. Intuition
7. Connection

Taking the awareness we have cultivated forward, we then open a deep creative flow, and finally we express our ideas and insights through the spoken and written word.

The actual Conscious Writing process is a series of specific conscious actions that enable us to transition from everyday mode into the present, aligned, and connected state of being we need for any kind of original creative work. Yet, we can take the principles and apply them in a more general way to have direct personal experience of this conscious approach to creative awakening.

Dive In

Instead of rushing straight into whatever creative work you're intending to do, take some time to follow these simple steps first:

1. Relax and Energize Your Body

Research shows that moving your body boosts your creativity. Depending on the time you have available, go for a walk, do some yoga, or simply spend a few minutes stretching and shaking out your physical body to release any tension and enhance the flow of energy. Inhabit your body fully, deepen your breathing, and enjoy feeling centered and grounded as a result.

2. Open Up Positive Emotion

Numerous studies have been done that correlate being in a positive mood with enhanced creativity. Essentially, this is because, when you're feeling happy, you're in an open and expanded state of being. So, remember a time when you felt joyful, grateful, and filled with love. Recreate those feelings now; place your hands over your heart; smile and flood your body with feel-good hormones.

3. Clear Space in Your Mind

If your mind is filled with the incessant chatter of what Buddhists call the "monkey mind," access to your true self and the essence of your true voice becomes blocked. Create space by sitting still with your eyes closed and focus your attention on the spaces between your thoughts. Initially, these may last only a fraction of a second; but, with practice, your ability to maintain awareness of the space instead of the thought stream will expand.

4. Connect with Your Core

The first three steps will lead you to feel a deeper sense of connection with yourself than might usually be the case. Take this one step further by turning your palms to face upward as a symbolic gesture of opening and receiving. Surrender your will to greater awareness beyond your everyday self and affirm your intention to be the vehicle through which your highest purpose will pour.

5. Express Yourself Freely

With practice and repetition, arriving at this point of readiness to explore your ideas and express your true voice freely and without judgment can be reached in a matter of moments. Whenever possible, immerse yourself more deeply and spend longer at each stage as the benefits are cumulative. The more you engage with this holistic approach, the greater your rewards will be.

Ultimately, who you become in the process of discovering and expressing your true voice is the greatest reward of all. From the perspective of Conscious Writing, this is the quintessence of who you are as you express yourself consciously and creatively in all areas of your life. Namaste.

Julia McCutchen is an intuitive mentor, the founder and creative director of the International Association of Conscious & Creative Writers (IACCW), and the author of Conscious Writing: Discover Your True Voice Through Mindfulness and More. A former publisher of spiritual and personal development books, a life-changing accident triggered a series of major quantum leaps in her spiritual awakening. Today, Julia's passion is to guide you to discover your true self and express your true voice on the page and in the world. Visit her websites: JuliaMc-Cutchen.com and iaccw.com

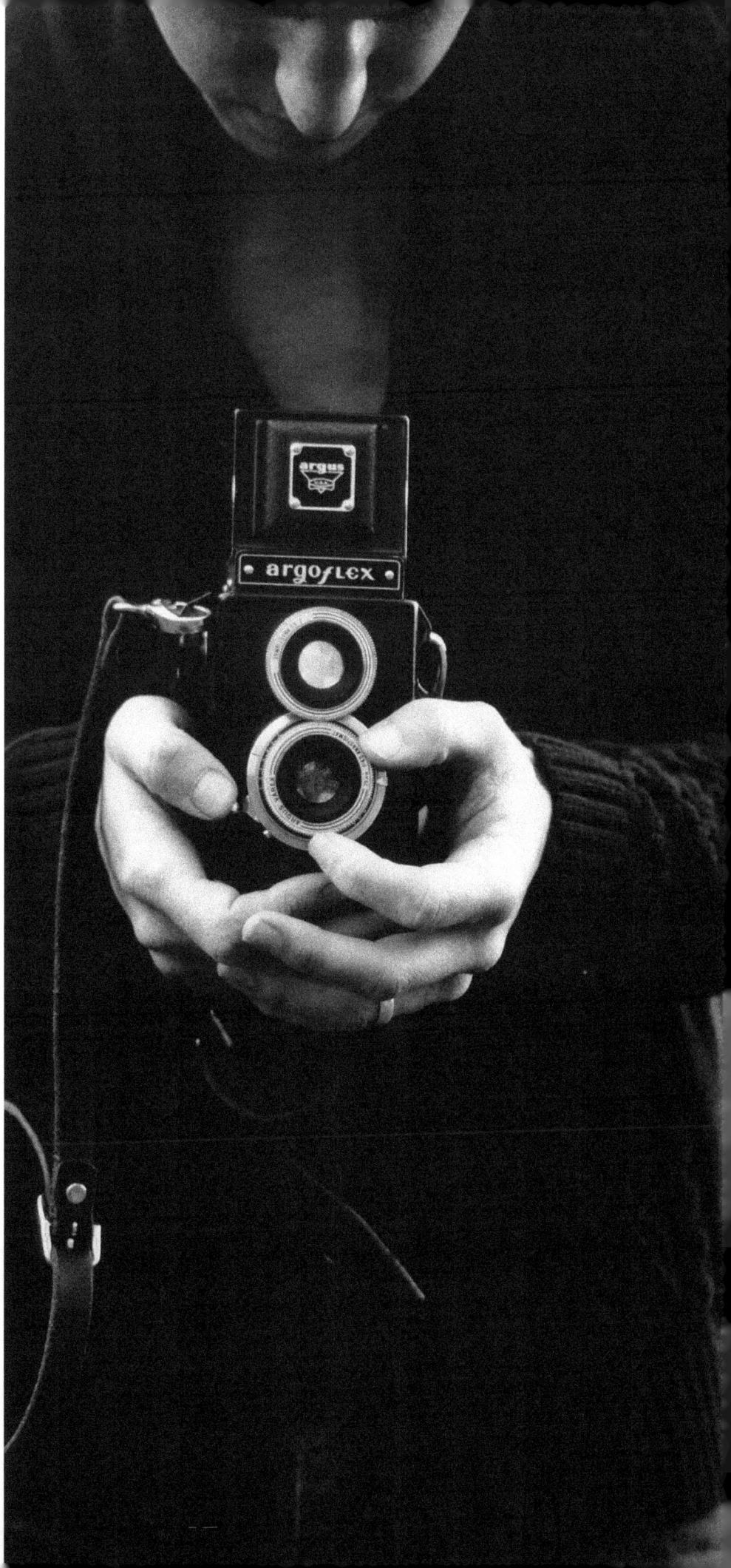

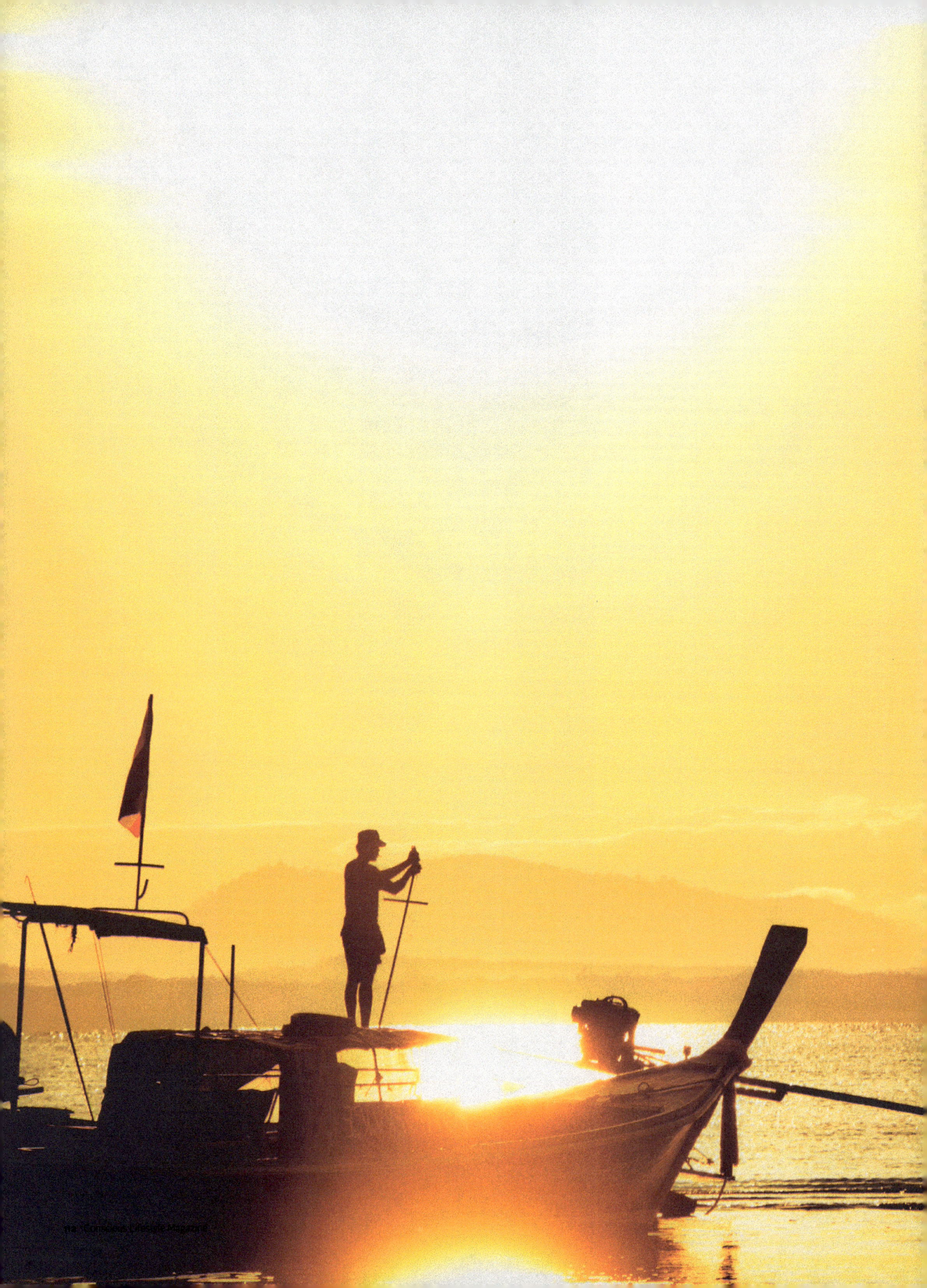

BALI

Adrift in the Indonesian archipelago of the
Northeastern Indian Ocean, Bali is an oasis of
meditative natural beauty, deeply spiritual island
culture and the raw power and intensity of Mother
Nature in an ancient dance with it all.

by ryan mandell

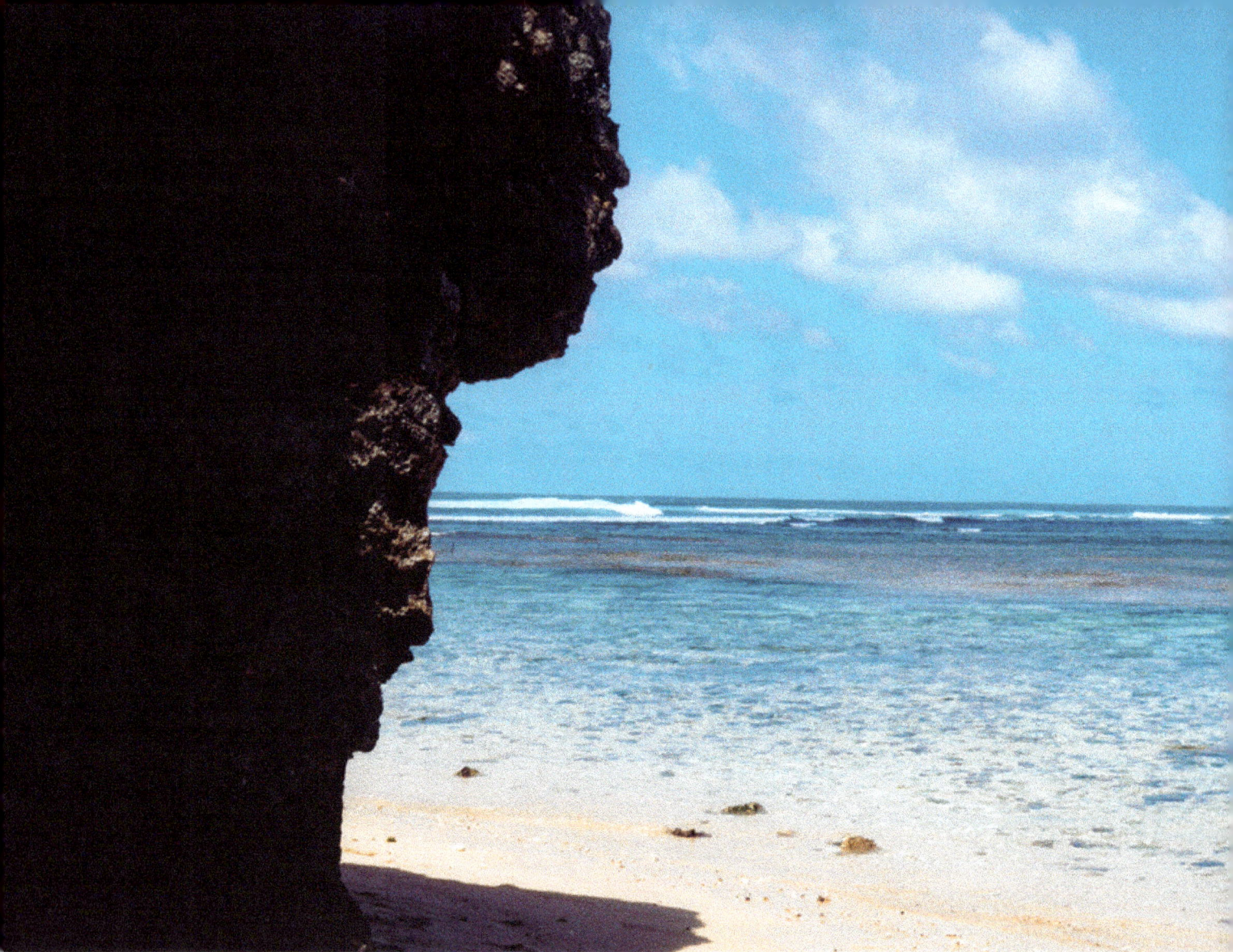

Bali is an elixir of gratitude, joy, healing, and freedom that embraces all life and the art of living richly and fully.

The island of Gods, the island of love—Bali is the watering hole for the soul. Hiding nothing from no one, the separations and connections of man and nature, and the interwoven nature of all life, are exposed for all to see. One is overwhelmed by the visceral beauty of nature, the beauty of humanity—and their respective shadows. Bali is a paradox, embodying both the yin and yang in all its machinations. Here, there is no gray area; unlike the veiled narrative of the rest of the world, here, we can definitively feel the divine and deepen our connection with its essence. In Bali, the eternal is easy to understand: you can hear the echo of our planet whispering, "We are here together."

The Balinese are often described as some of the warmest people on the planet. Ingrained into the culture and land itself is a spirit that uplifts its people in both synchronistic and unexpected ways. The island's mystical nature surprises visitors with revelations and clarity by encouraging that which needs

to unfold to blossom. Tens of thousands of people fly into Bali's international airport everyday, some yearn to escape western culture and it's overly rational and ego-driven undertones, some to catch the perfect wave, and others simply to find some peace and quiet with a soul-nourishing ocean view and sacred monkeys swinging through the trees. Whatever your motivation, Bali is an elixir of gratitude, joy, healing, and freedom that embraces all life and the art of living richly and fully.

Kuta

As the airplane enters the international airport, brightly colored boats and swelling waves circulate in the surrounding electric blue Indian Ocean. Originally a favorite destination among surfers due to its long beaches and mind-bending reef breaks, Kuta is now the largest tourist hub in Bali. As such, it is very congested with traffic, tourists, and local peoples—for this reason I would not recom-

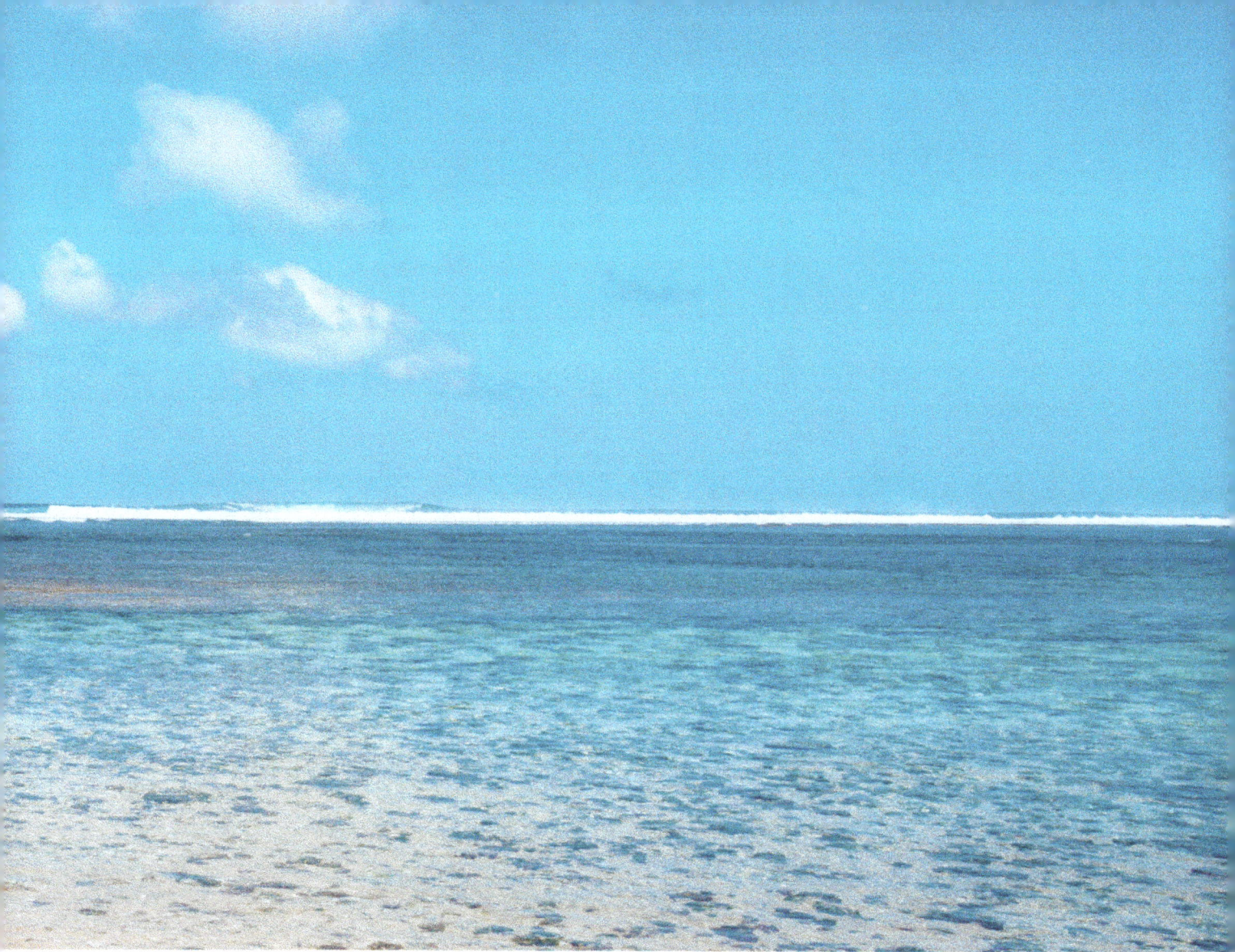

mend spending more than a few days here at most, but with that being said there are some very fun things to do. Jalan Legian is the main street that runs from north to south Kuta and through Seminyak. It is full of shops, hotels, restaurants, bars, and nightclubs, if that's your kind of thing. Sky Garden is the most famous club (or infamous, depending on who you ask), known for attracting famous DJs from around the world. If you decide to indulge, there are many spas that offer healing treatments for a fraction of the cost of western establishments to soothe the mind and body the morning after. Of course one could also just as easily grab a waiting boatman off the beach for a trip out to Kuta Reef to let the light in with a solid morning surf session. Compared to the rest of Bali, Kuta is rambunctious—although the city can be intense at times, it's balanced by the distinctly spiritual overtones of the Balinese people. You can catch glimpses of their offerings to the gods, *canang sari*, nearly everywhere you go,

which is a bamboo leaf tied up with incense and colorful food.

Canggu

Canggu could theoretically be included in the Kuta section as it is a northern suburb of the city, however, it's nothing like Kuta proper. If you decide to go, I'd recommend heading out to Echo beach. One word of advice: don't step on the coral—first of all, it's sharp and second, it's alive. Canggu has the relaxed atmosphere of the Bukit Peninsula, but is more central with plenty of accommodations and restaurants, like the Betelnut Café, serving up organic Indonesian and western fare. Lining the beach, which happens to have great surf as well, you'll also find various grills serving fresh caught fish for a princely sum of about $6. If you have to spend a night or two close to the airport for any reason, this is the place to do it rather than stay in Kuta proper. It's got a far more relaxed vibe and reflects the more soulful nature of Bali without having to

This is a place to let go and simply be present with the abundance of Mother Nature and the infinite beauty of life itself.

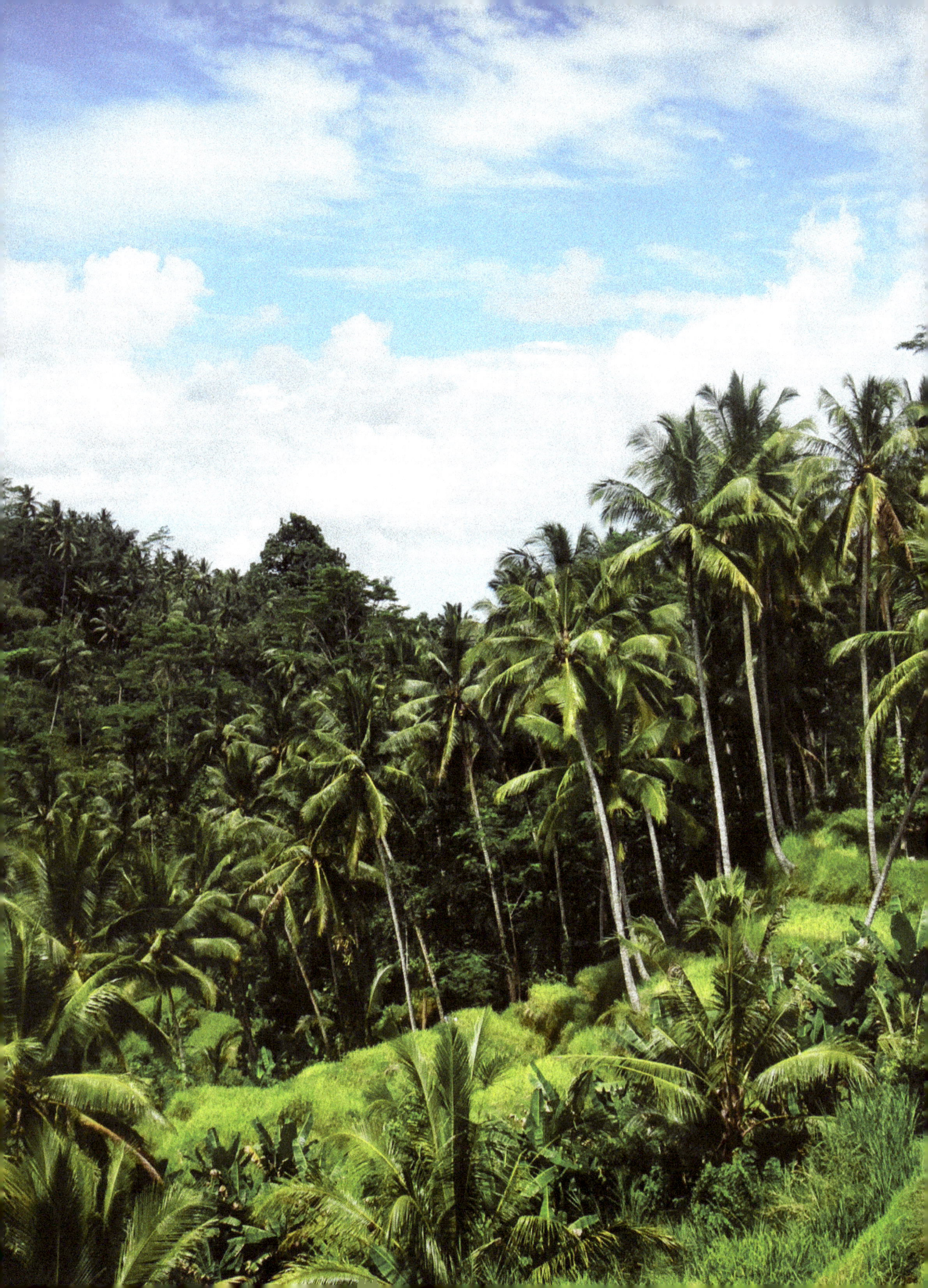

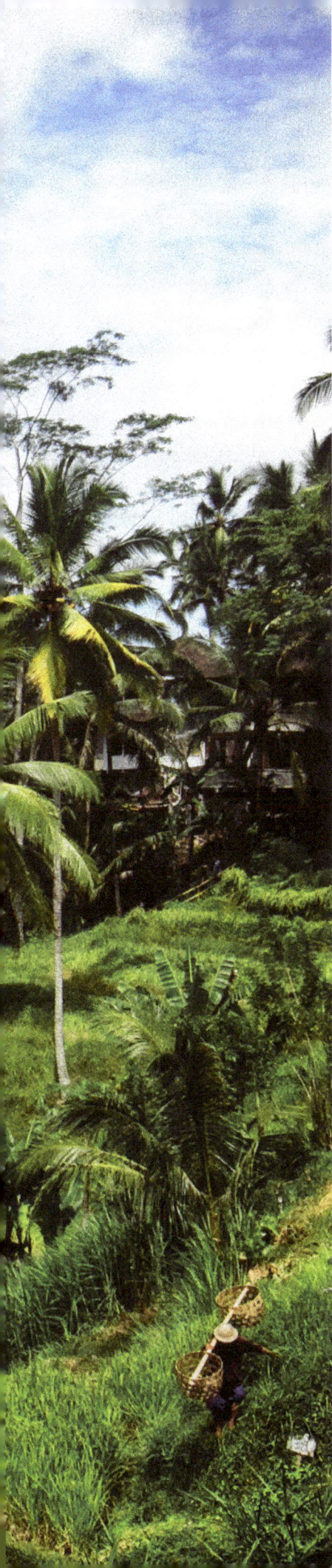

travel to more remote parts of the island.

Lembongan

To truly experience the essence of Bali, one should distance themselves from Kuta and the crowds, and there are few places better to do that than Lembongan, a small island off the coast of the Bali mainland that is just a quick 30-minute boat ride away. Lembongan is a place out of time, where time seems to slow down and everything non-essential simply melts away. There is enough of a town, and a handful of restaurants and hotels to give comfort to travelers, but other than that there is not much else to do, save for letting yourself get lost in the stunning natural beauty of the jungles, reefs, and crystal blue waters. This is a place to let go and simply be present with the abundance of Mother Nature and the infinite beauty of life itself. Upon arrival to the island, you are overwhelmed with panoramic views of craggy cliffs jutting out over the sea in an endless dramatic clash with incoming Indian Ocean swells that send mountains of explosive white water pluming into the air. At low tide, the boats coast to the shore floating delicately in the glass-like water, their bottoms mere inches above the sand, kelp, and coral.

To get a full taste of the mind-body-spirit synthesis that Bali embodies, I recommend booking Rick Cowley's Vision Quest Bali retreat, which is a 7-day holistic adventure combining yoga, meditation, scooter riding, surfing, snorkeling, and cliff jumping at the phenomenally beautiful blue lagoon. We nestled in a small bungalow-style homestay, replete with an infinity pool and fully staffed restaurant, on a cliff overlooking the heaving ocean swells. Each night during high tide you could feel the power of the waves reverberate throughout the bungalows as they smashed against the rocks below. The mornings revealed brightly colored boats beached on the vibrant coral reefs by low tide. Riding my battered Suzuki scooter along the dusty dirt roads and towering cable bridges on the

> Lembongan is a place out of time, where time seems to slow down and everything non-essential simply melts away.

Ubud is the crown jewel of conscious travel in Bali. Lush green and mind-bogglingly gorgeous.

return trip to the mainland, I dropped into a new level of connectedness with the essence of who I truly was, the Vision Quest weaving the spirit of Bali even deeper into my soul.

If you are looking for an incredibly deep transformational experience beyond the normal fare of yoga and meditation retreats, check out Oceans Health Retreat run by Kerri Blake, a masterful healer, coach and journey work facilitator known worldwide for her ability to clear decades of emotional blocks in an incredibly short period of time.

Uluwatu

About an hour south of Kuta, which is a world away in Bali, is the Bukit Peninsula. The west side is home to the beautiful beaches of Bingin Beach, Jimbaran, Uluwatu, and Padang Padang. The edges of the peninsula are cradled in soaring, vine-covered cliffs that tower over the powder white coral sand beaches below. This is the Bali that everyone dreams about... the almost painfully beautiful and romantic beaches that lure countless travelers from every corner of the globe. Panoramic views of endlessly long stretches of rainbow coral reefs and limestone cliffs have hypnotized visitors for millennia. In the evening you are rewarded with glowing golden sunsets that paint the water with a rich orange sheen. They are best enjoyed with a sampling of the exotic local fruit juices, ranging from vibrantly pink, fresh-blended watermelon juice to nutrient-rich young coconut water and everything in between. This is also the perfect time to lose yourself in meditation—shutting off the critical faculties of the mind to simply sit back and bask in the beauty of it all.

Bingin Beach is a favorite of backpackers and nomads because of the abundance of cheap yet comfortable accommodations overlooking the beach. Homestays line the vertical cliffs; stay at the top if you want a good view or at the bottom if you want to be close to the beach and avoid the long treacherous hike up the unruly stairs. During the day, surfers play amongst the perfect waves, children swim in the tide pools, and their parents relax on the coral sand beaches. There are three accessible surf breaks from Bingin Beach: Bingin Reef, Impossibles, and Dreamlands. Bali is known worldwide for it's near-perfect, mind-bending surf, but if you're a beginner there are plenty of surf schools to get you started in a more mellow setting. And if surfing isn't your thing, then you can still use the undulating rhythm of the waves to guide yourself into deep states of meditation and relaxation.

At night, several beachfront restaurants prepare freshly caught fish over glowing hot coals and coconut husks for visitors to enjoy on the moonlit sands. This is the perfect way to wind down after a day spent with friends hiking up and down the hundreds of stairs lining the towering cliffs after a mind-blowing surf or snorkeling session. A handful of the restaurants are strictly vegan as well, so all palettes are well cared for. If you are staying in the area for any length of time, we recommend the Temple Lodge, a gorgeous, conscious yoga and surfing retreat center featuring organic Ayurvedic and macrobiotic-inspired meals with stunning views.

Ubud

Ubud is the crown jewel of conscious travel in Bali. Lush green and mind-bogglingly gorgeous, Ubud is home to many soul-nourishing spiritual experiences, retreats and restaurants, and a haven for seekers worldwide. If you find yourself in the area, there are a few seminal things that are not to be missed:

Pura Goa Gajah

Translated as the elephant cave temple, this structure was originally built in the 9th century and transports visitors back in time to when Indonesia was nothing more than a primal, remote, mystical jungle harboring deeply spiritual and aware native people.

High Priestess Water Purification Ceremony

Ida Resi Alit, a Balinese High Priestess, conducts special purification ceremonies using sacred, blessed water in the remote village

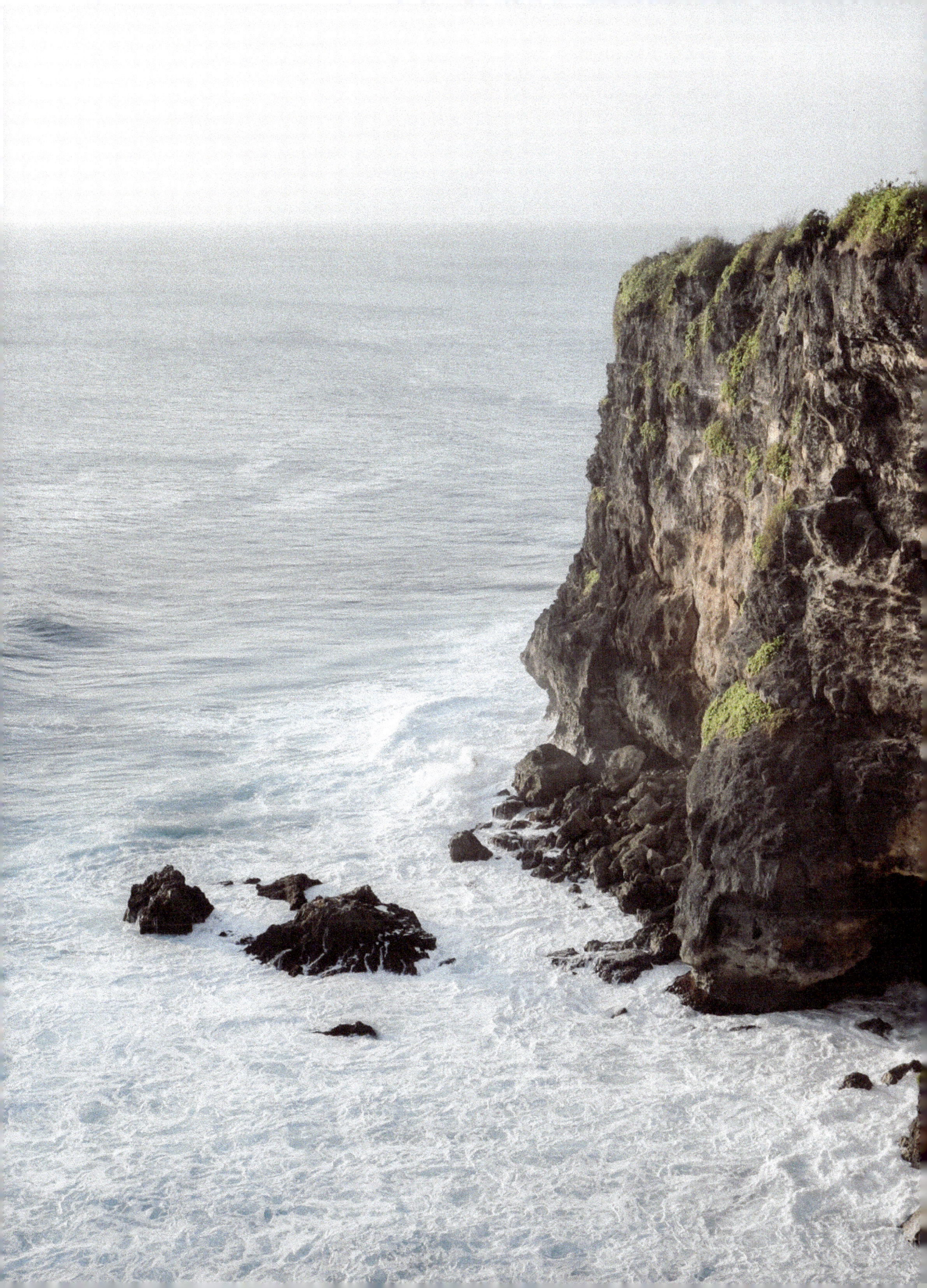

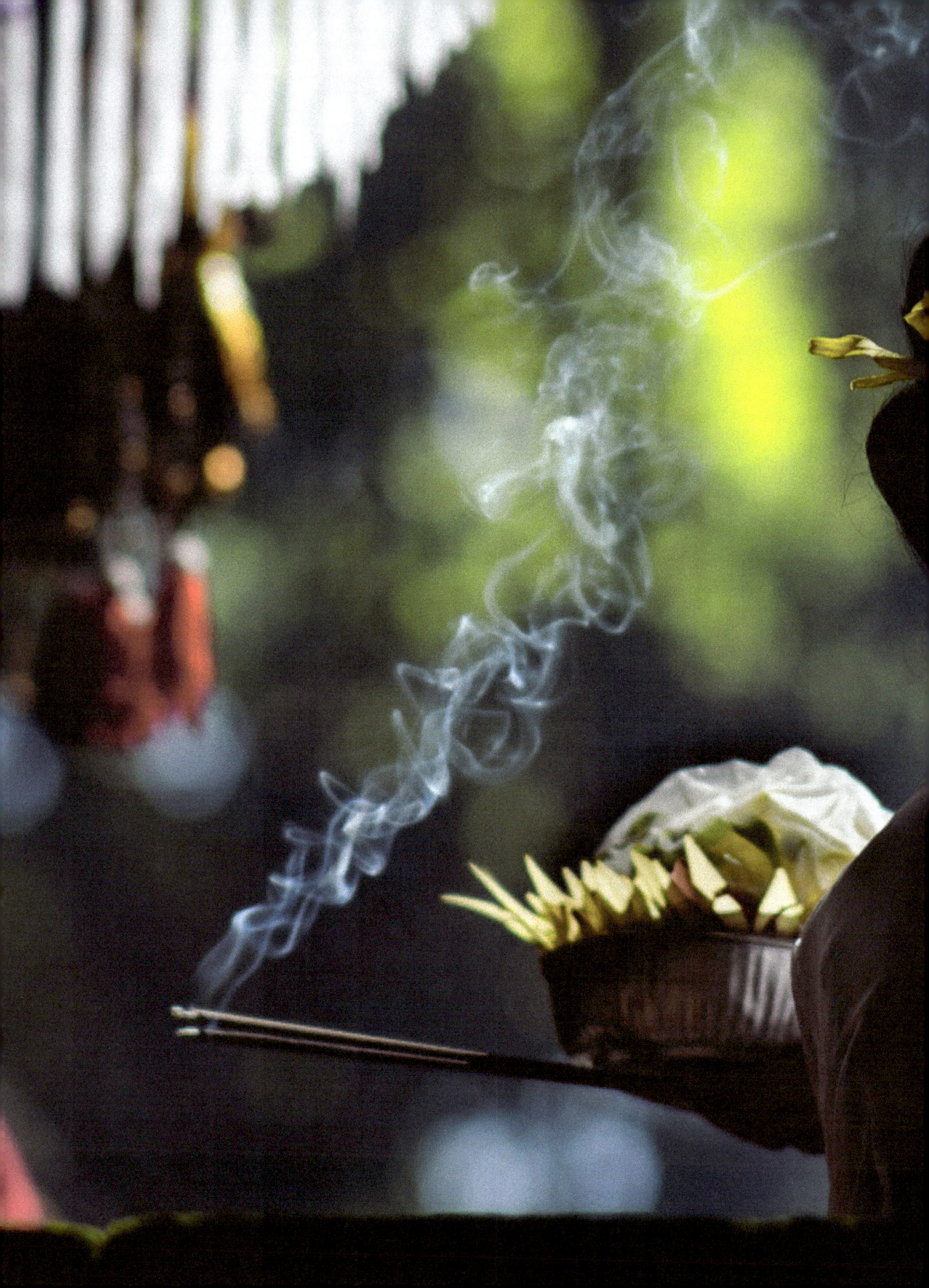

Demulih, if you can find her. The highly symbolic ritual combines, prayer, intention and mindfulness, and is intended to purify the mind, body and spirit, giving seekers a taste of the deep, traditional spiritual culture still running strong in Bali.

Jamie Lu Sound Healing Experience

Jamie is a gifted intuitive healer utilizing a variety of methods, including touch, sound, and energy work to induce transformation and balance on every level of the mind, body and spirit. She is world-renowned for working with difficult illnesses and diseases, after healing herself from a heart condition and Hashimoto's disease at age 24. Be sure to drop in for one of her deeply nourishing and revitalizing sound healings, personalized to your needs.

In recent years countless raw food cafés and juice bars have sprung up in Ubud, and the area has traditionally been a hotbed for healers, meditators, yogis, and similar ilk. There are a number of retreats and conscious accommodations, making this an area to spend some time in if this is how you like to travel.

Surrounding the city are breathtaking rice terraces, which are a great place to catch a sunset and spend some time in silent contemplation. Walking through and around the terraces one starts to feel as if in a maze of dreamlike beauty, immersed in the spirit of the rice paddies. The symbiotic relationship between man and nature, as well as the abundance of nature flourishing all around you, is an experience that is not to be missed and is a microcosm of Bali as a whole.

Ryan Mandell is a writer, musician, surfer, yogi, and artist. He developed an early interest in spirituality as a child finding himself strongly drawn to the eastern religions of Buddhism and Hinduism. Visit his website: getatpookie.bandcamp.com

The highly symbolic ritual combines, prayer, intention and mindfulness, and is intended to purify the mind, body and spirit.

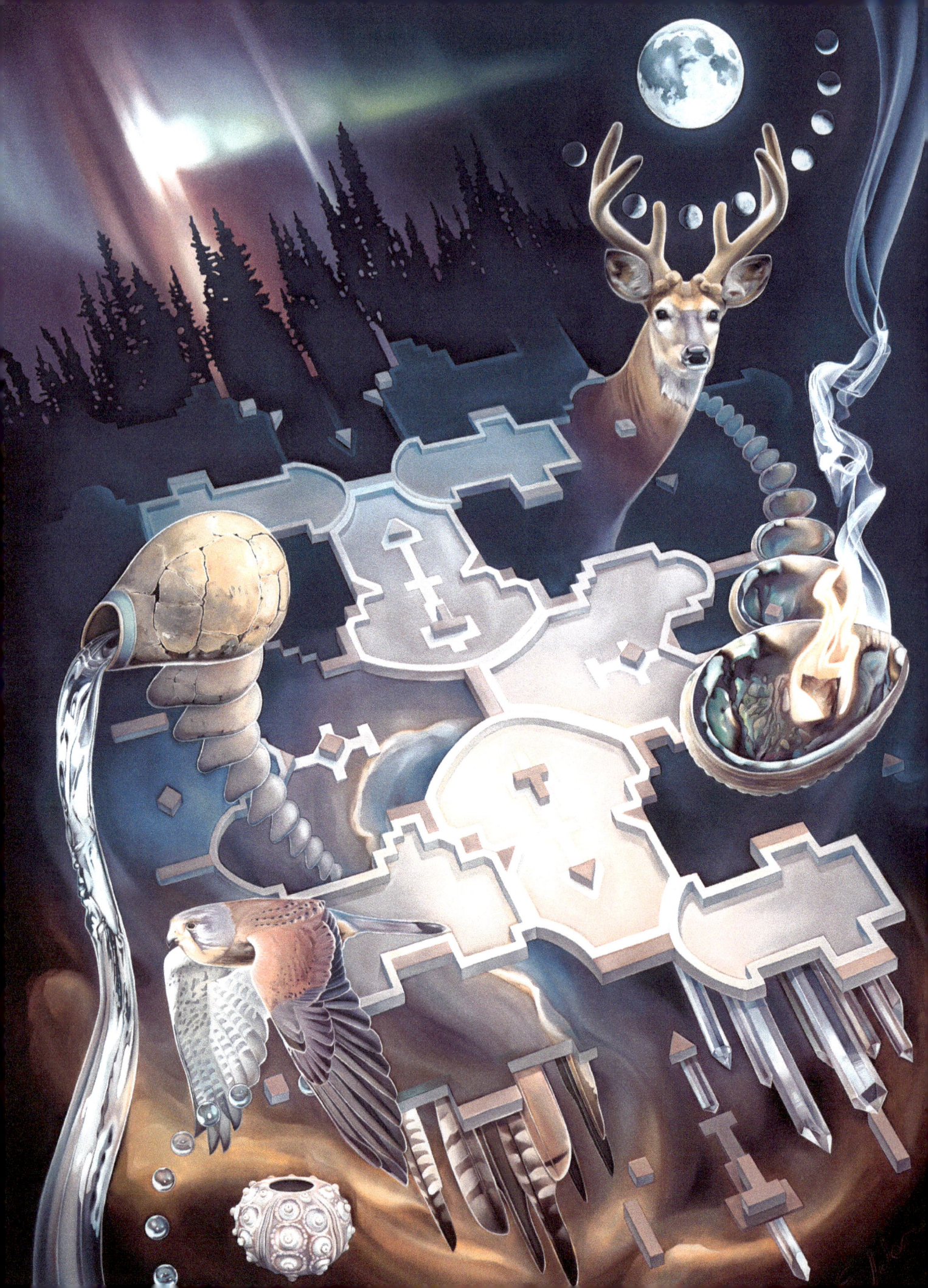

Mystical Realities: The Art of Collin Elder

There's something distinctly primal but also simultaneously spiritual about Collin Elder's evocative paintings. Shamanically blending dreamlike machinations of the human figure and mind with the natural world, they reveal themselves in layers—upon closer inspection sacred geometries and fractals emerge from the abstractions alongside synergies of both animal and human forms, enmeshed in the fabric of their ecological origins. And that's intentional on both an actualized and philosophical level: Collin's work, in his own words, is meant to explore the "depths of our links with the non-human, and hopefully connect their remembering with the health of our human community."

With a background in conservation and a degree in wildlife biology, his work is "an effort to evoke a vivid sense of direct experience." To essentially reconnect us with that which has been lost in our transition from an agrarian to technological society. His vibrant paintings pierce directly into the heart and rekindle forgotten aspects of the soul, reconnecting us to the mystical realities just out-side our everyday awareness. They encourage us to transcend the "idea of looking through our investigations, classifications, sciences and technologies, into active, subjective participation with an integral, holistic and mysterious ecosystem."

I believe there is a deeper message in his work—that everything is one. That the separations we believe exist between ourselves and our environment are simply figments of our misperception. After all, at the sub-atomic level, everything is made of the same cosmic matter—electrons, protons, neutrons, all arranged in an infinite variety of shapes, colors and sizes. Where then does one thing end and the next begin? What separates the essence of you from the essence of a tree, or a wolf, or a star, or anything else for that matter? Nothing, it seems. And in that sense, perhaps Collin's paintings are a much more accurate reflection of the true nature of reality than we let ourselves believe...

Learn more at: collinelder.com

> I believe there is a deeper message in his work—that everything is one.

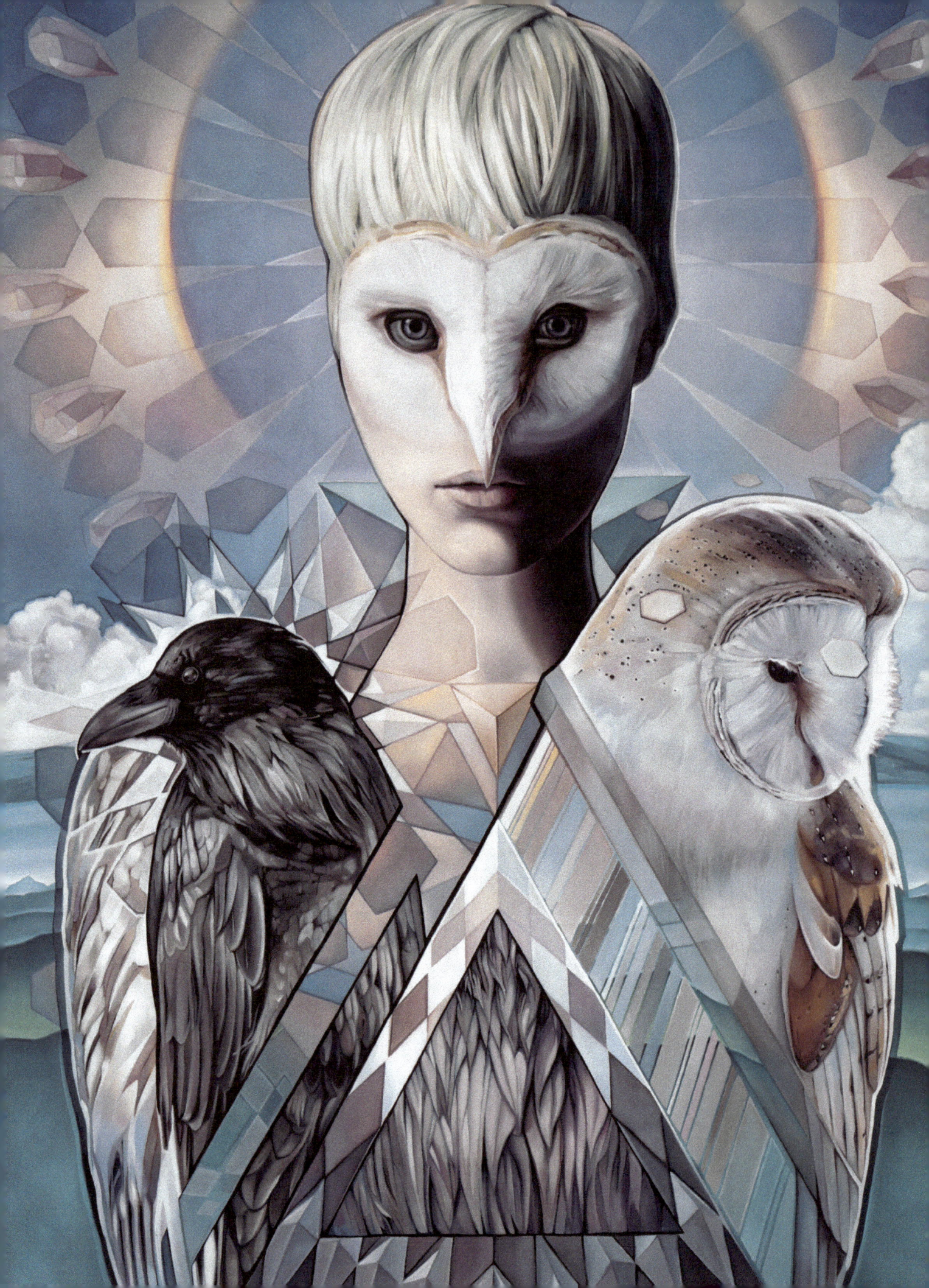

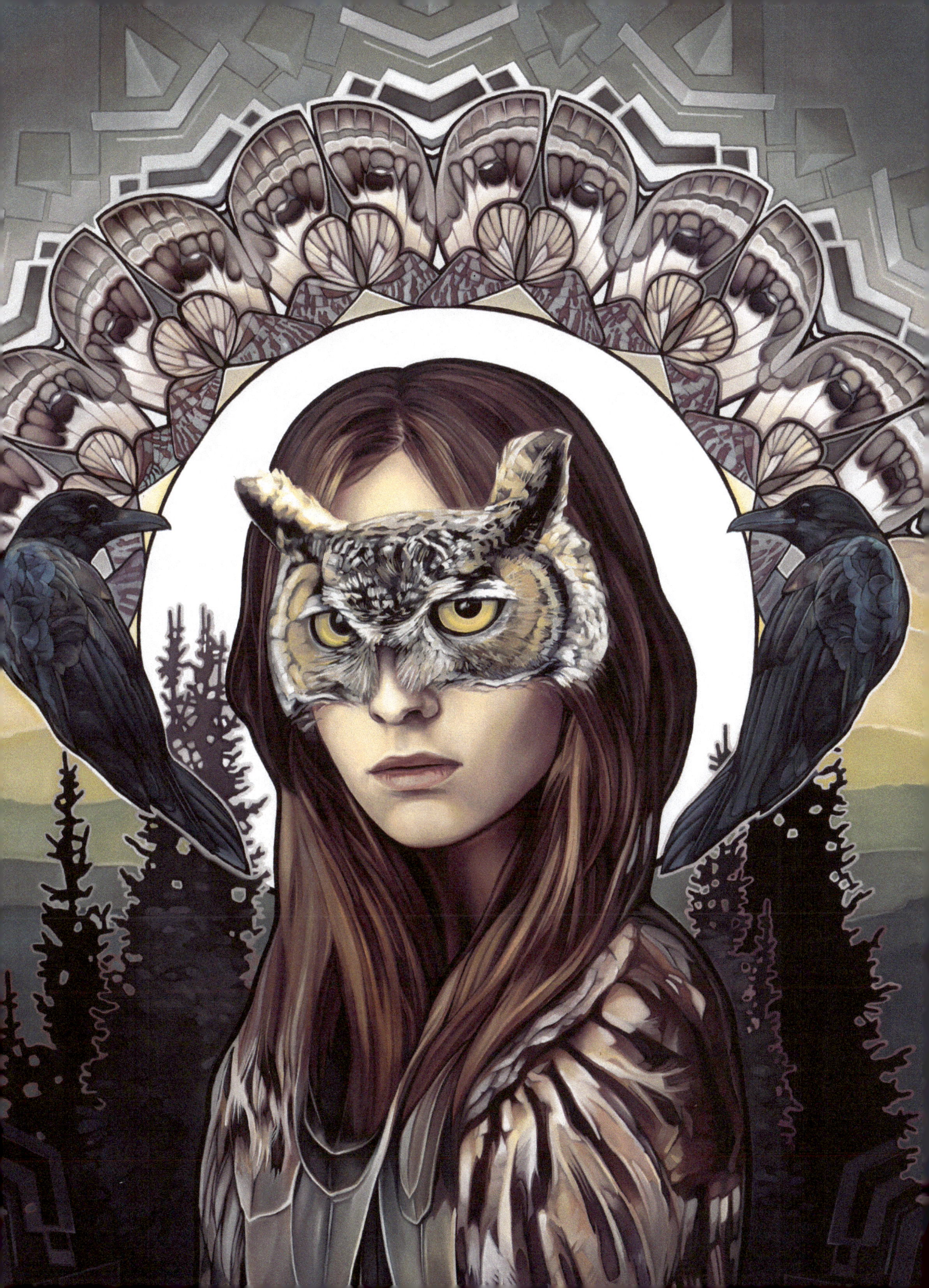

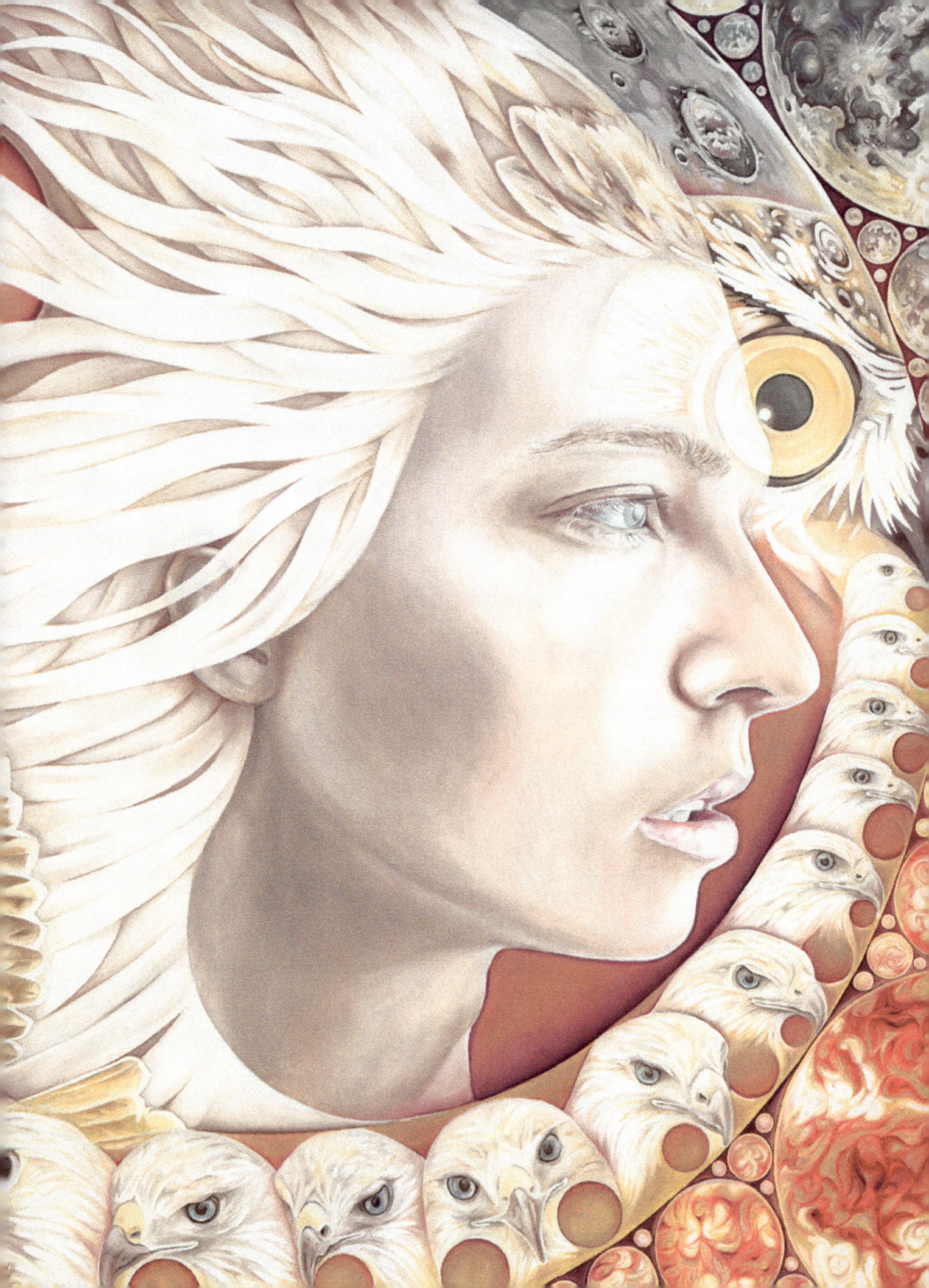

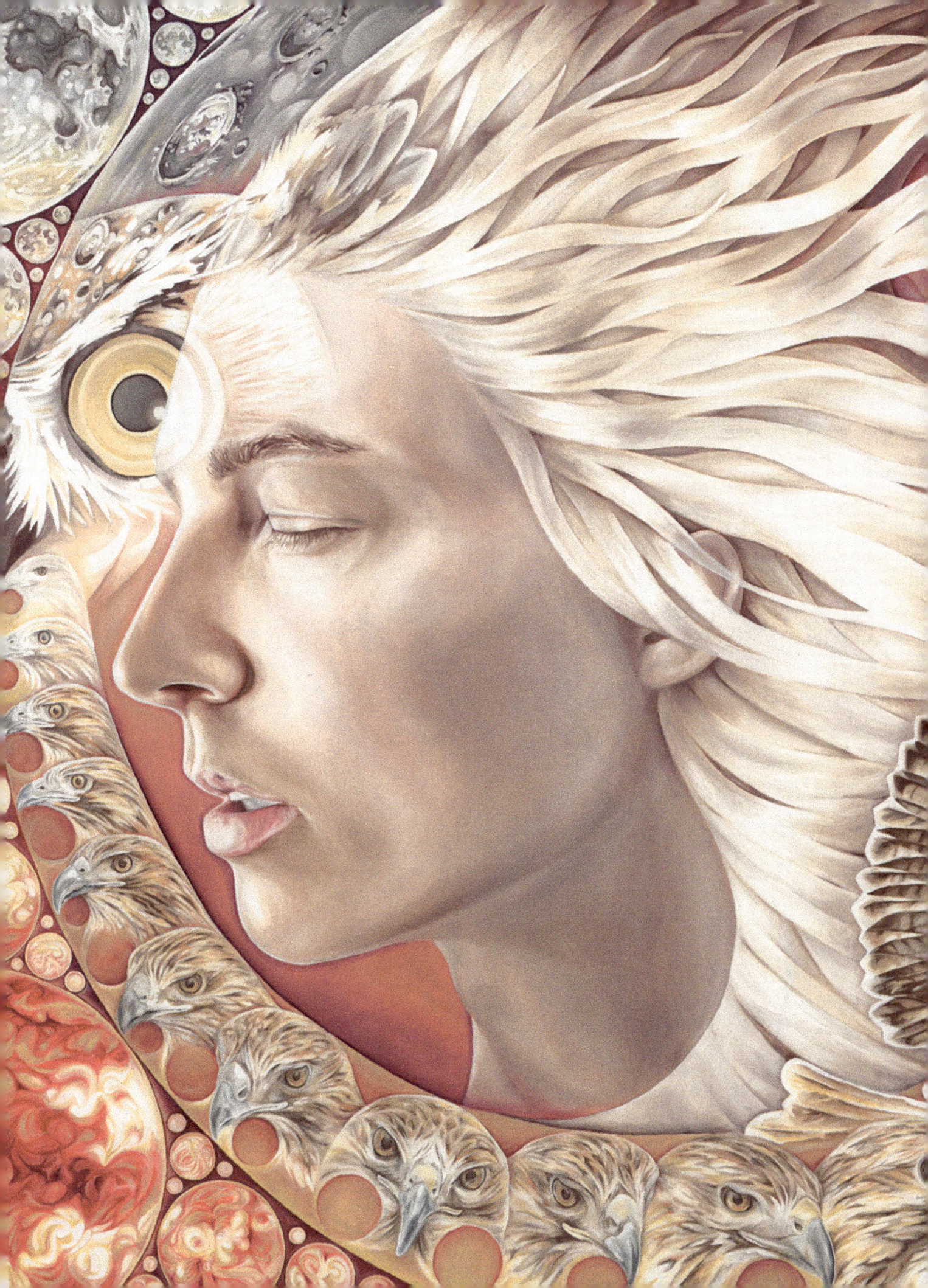

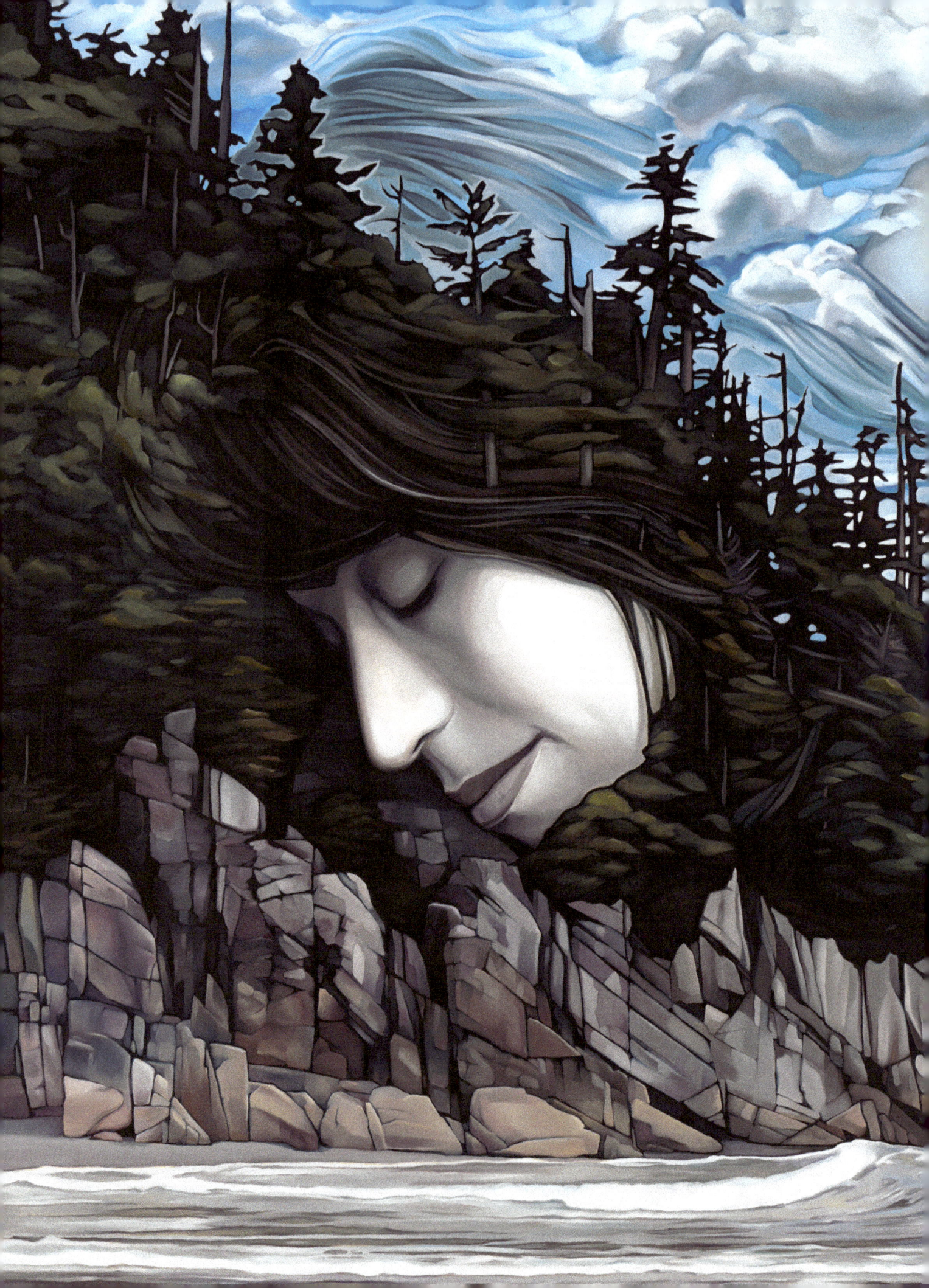

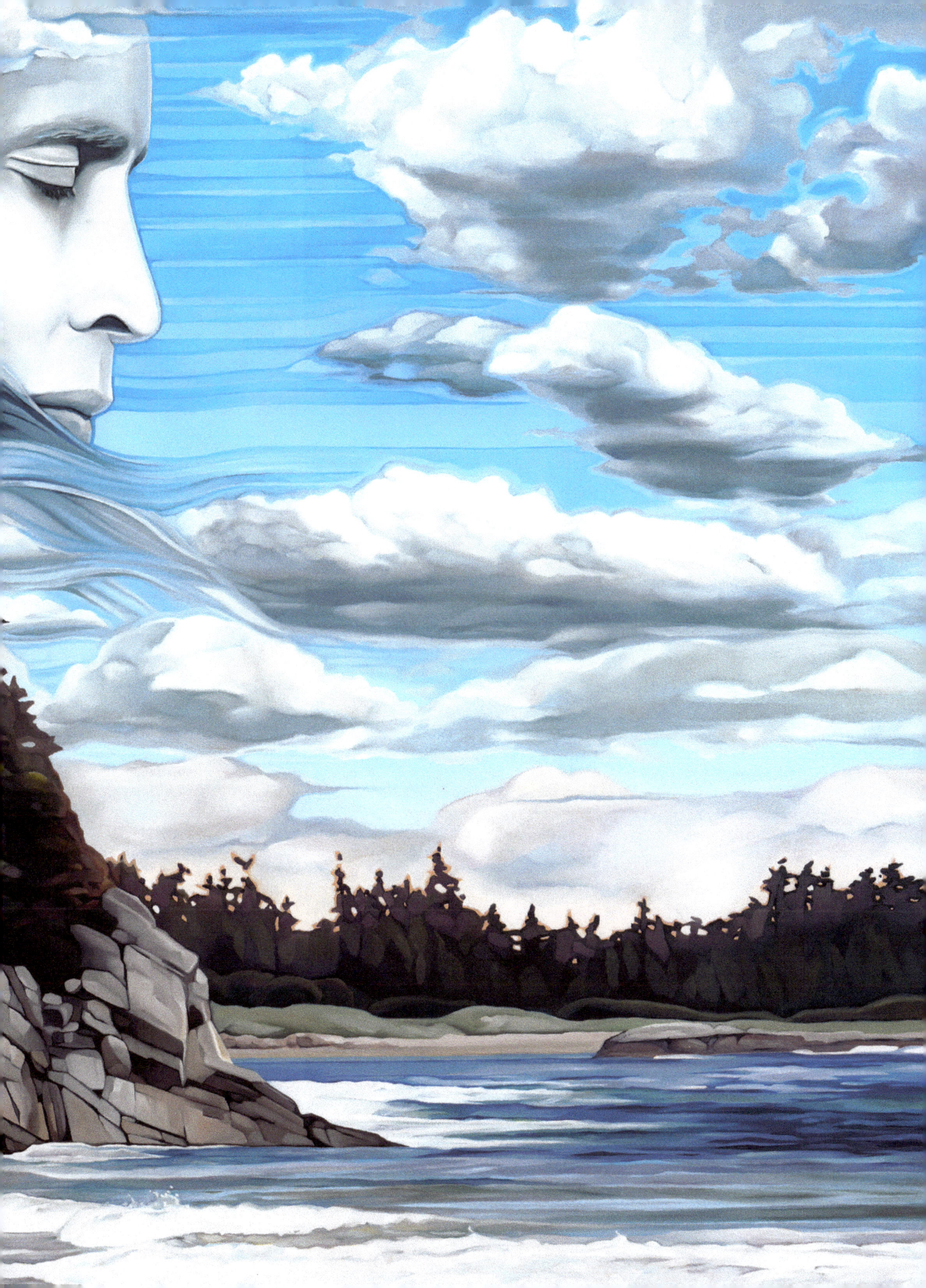

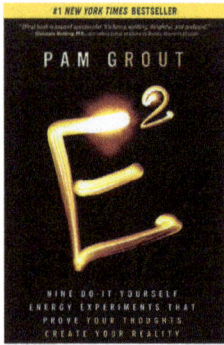

E-SQUARED: NINE DO-IT-YOURSELF ENERGY EXPERIMENTS THAT PROVE YOUR THOUGHTS CREATE YOUR REALITY
Pam Grout, Hay House

E-Squared could best be described as a lab manual with simple experiments to prove once and for all that reality is malleable, that consciousness trumps matter, and that you shape your life with your mind. Rather than take it on faith, you are invited to conduct nine 48-hour experiments to prove there really is a positive, loving, totally hip force in the universe. The experiments, each of which can be conducted with absolutely no money and very little time expenditure, demonstrate that spiritual principles are as dependable as gravity, as *consistent* as Newton's laws of motion.

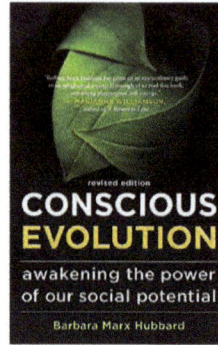

CONSCIOUS EVOLUTION: AWAKENING THE POWER OF OUR SOCIAL POTENTIAL
Barbara Marx Hubbard, New World Library

With her clear-eyed, inspiring, and sweeping vision of a possible global renaissance in the new millennium, Hubbard shows us that our current crises are not the precursors of an apocalypse but the natural birth pains of an awakened, universal humanity. In this edition of *Conscious Evolution*, Barbara carries us beyond the human potential movement into the social potential movement. She describes a holistic social architecture to enhance and connect social innovations that are now evolving our world toward social synergy, interconnectivity, and spirit-based compassion for all.

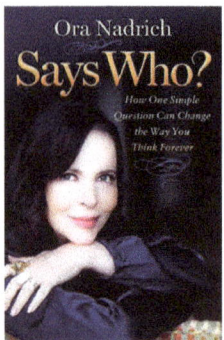

SAYS WHO? HOW ONE SIMPLE QUESTION CAN CHANGE THE WAY YOU THINK FOREVER
Ora Nadrich, Morgan James Publishing

Many of the obstacles people face are the result of their own negative thoughts holding them back. And often those thoughts don't even originate within them; they're the ideas or opinions of someone else—a critical parent or angry spouse—which they believe without questioning to see if they're even real or true. Since thoughts and beliefs interact to influence behavior, negative thoughts are dangerous things to leave unchecked. You must question and challenge them. *Says Who?* shows us how with a simple, effective process that can be used daily.

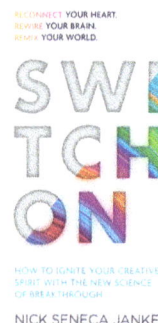

SWITCH ON: UNLEASH YOUR CREATIVITY AND THRIVE WITH THE NEW SCIENCE & SPIRIT OF BREAKTHROUGH
Nick Seneca Jankel, Watkins

Switch On presents a compelling answer to one of the most pressing questions we face today: How do we as individuals, and our world as a whole, thrive? Backed in science and inspired by age-old wisdom, the answer coalesces 20 years of research and experience at the forefront of personal, social and corporate change. The result is Breakthrough Biodynamics, a groundbreaking fusion of the latest neuroscience, years of evolution, ancient traditions, practical philosophy, and powerful tools for making transformation happen.

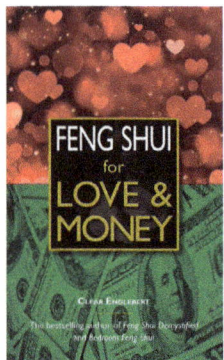

FENG SHUI FOR LOVE & MONEY
Clear Englebert, Watermark Publishing

Money can't buy you love, but feng shui can help you attract both. *Feng Shui for Love & Money* offers practical solutions for enhancing your bank account and your relationships. This feng shui guide from bestselling author and feng shui consultant Clear Englebert offers easy-to-follow advice for promoting prosperity and attracting and enhancing relationships. Real life examples and simple illustrations are included throughout the book, which aid in visualizing feng shui problem situations and the placement of objects to remedy them.

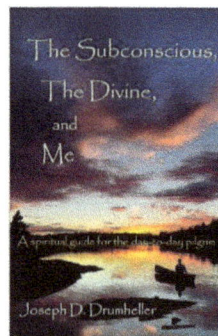

THE SUBCONSCIOUS, THE DIVINE AND ME: A SPIRITUAL GUIDE FOR THE DAY-TO-DAY PILGRIM
Joseph Drumheller, Pine Winds Press

A profound introduction to the inner workings of the subconscious mind, energy healing and spirituality. Through six succinct and brilliant lessons certified hypnotherapist and spiritual seeker, Joseph Drumheller, imbues the knowledge and guidance needed to move from pain and suffering to empowerment and freedom. Each of the six lessons include rich stories and practical exercises, bringing you ever closer to healing and awakening, and restoring your power to create positive transformation in your life.

www.ingramcontent.com/pod-product-compliance
Lightning Source LLC
Chambersburg PA
CBHW051612030426

42334CB00035B/3498